THE ARTHRITIS CURE FITNESS SOLUTION

THE ARTHRITIS CURE FITNESS SOLUTION

by Brenda D. Adderly, M.H.A., and Chanteil Miller, C.P.F.T.

LifeLine
Press

An Eagle Publishing Company • Washington, DC

Library of Congress Cataloging-in-Publication Data

Adderly, Brenda.
    The arthritis cure fitness solution / by Brenda Adderly and Chanteil Miller.
        p. cm.
    Includes bibliographical references and index.
    ISBN 0–89526–359–9 (alk. paper)
    1. Arthritis—Exercise therapy. I. Miller, Chanteil. II. Title.
    RC933.A34 1999
    616.7'22062—dc21   98–55567
                                                                             CIP

Published in the United States by
LifeLine Press
An Eagle Publishing Company
One Massachusetts Avenue, NW
Washington, DC 20001

Distributed to the trade by
National Book Network
4720-A Boston Way
Lanham, MD 20706

Printed on acid-free paper.
Manufactured in the United States of America

BOOK DESIGN BY MARJA WALKER
SET IN GARAMOND THREE

10 9 8 7 6 5 4 3 2 1

Books are available in quantity for promotional or premium use. Write to Director of Special Sales, LifeLine Press, One Massachusetts Avenue, NW, Washington, DC 20001, for information on discounts and terms or call (202) 216-0600.

CONTENTS

ACKNOWLEDGMENTS

I'd like to acknowledge the contributions of those who guided us through the development and successful completion of this project—Jeff Still and Howard Cohl at Affinity Communications, and a special thanks to Mari Florence.

— *Brenda Adderly*

I extend a heartfelt thank you to the many wonderful people associated with the publishing company whose patience, diligence, and insight has allowed me the opportunity to be a part of the solution.

— *Chanteil Miller*

CHAPTER ONE

Beginning Your Journey to Fitness

*"The first secret you should know about perfect health is that
you have to choose it. You can only be as healthy as you think
it is possible to be. Perfect health is no mere 5 or 10 percent
improvement over good health. It involves a total shift in per-
spective which makes disease and infirm old age unacceptable."*

—DEEPAK CHOPRA, PERFECT HEALTH

BARBARA WAS AN ACTIVE WOMAN who exercised regularly
and considered herself athletic as well as attractive. After experiencing some health problems resulting in thyroid surgery, she gained a
considerable amount of weight and was unable to lose it. Then she
began to experience pain in her knees. Within a few years, the pain
spread to her hands and spine, and was so debilitating that she
rarely exercised and consequently, gained even more weight.
Barbara's legs, which were once long and shapely, now looked dis-
figured. Barbara went to her doctor and was diagnosed with
osteoarthritis (OA).

"I cannot tell you how much having this disease has impacted me
and every single thing I do in my life," says Barbara, who is in her
fifties. "There have been times when the pain was so bad that I resis-
ted even getting up in the middle of the night for a glass of water....
It's tarnished my sense of well being, my sense of being young and
alive.... It [has] colored every life experience."

Then Barbara discovered water aerobics. She dedicated herself to
a three-day-a-week routine and, after six weeks, found complete
relief. "I woke up one day and said to my husband, 'I've been cured!'
And I really felt as though I was."

Unfortunately Barbara's work schedule changed and she could no
longer find time to go to the pool. After a few months the pain,

IMPROVE YOUR LIFE

To improve the quality of your life, you may have to make some lifestyle changes. That may include committing to an exercise program for the first time; releasing anger; embracing your power; finding or recommitting to a spiritual path; and taking responsibility for how you feel physically and emotionally. Ultimately, it means recognizing that you are choosing the life you live.

stiffness, and depression returned. And according to Barbara, "It hurt too much to exercise."

But now she's taking Osteo-Bi-Flex, the patented formula of glucosamine and chondroitin supplements, watching her diet, and has replaced water aerobics with walking. "...[S]ince I've been taking these supplements, life is so much more manageable.... Now I can walk, and maybe I'll be able to lose some weight...."

Barbara is on the road to being symptom-free once again. Her's is a success story. She is an exemplary member of the Arthritis Cure Fitness Team.

You can be, too! It *is* possible to feel good again.

By beginning the new Arthritis Cure Fitness Plan you will be adding a new dimension to improving your health. You will be on the road to enhanced health and increased vitality even though your life has been affected by arthritis.

WHAT IS ARTHRITIS?

The term "arthritis" refers to more than one hundred different conditions from simple swelling of the joints to fibromyalgia to lupus to bursitis. These conditions are always lumped together and called "arthritis" because they are all related to joints, muscles, tendons, ligaments, or bursa, and symptoms of the conditions are similar—usually manifesting as pain, inflammation, and limited joint movement. The Arthritis Cure Fitness Plan focuses on alleviating osteoarthritis, which is the most common form of arthritis that affects the joints. Recent studies show that approximately 10 percent of all people over age sixty-five experience pain related to osteoarthritis.[1]

Right now exercise may seem daunting to your mind and body, but be encouraged that the physical and mental health benefits will be a stronger, more flexible you.

OA OF THE KNEE? THE EVIDENCE SHOWS EXERCISE IS KEY

"Osteoarthritis patients who did aerobic exercises for 30 to 45 minutes three times a week were found to have such a reduction in pain that knee-replacement surgery was postponed possibly for years. Strengthened muscles around the knee joint tends to stabilize it with the resultant reduction in pain."

— *Prevention Magazine, May 1997*

"On completion of our [group exercise] study, more than 90 percent of the pain and physical function scores demonstrated significant improvements [in the patients with OA] without increases in medication, use of walking aids, or fatigue. The study suggests that [exercise] can reduce pain, increase physical function, and objective gait measures in subjects with osteoarthritis of the knee."

— *Physiotherapy Research International, 1997*

"People could prevent osteoarthritis simply by doing some simple exercises to keep their quadriceps in good shape. [Researchers] found that many of [the patients with OA] had weak quadriceps whether they felt pain or not... findings suggest that regular exercise to keep the quadriceps strong may help slow or prevent knee joint degeneration. By strengthening the quadriceps, people who already have osteoarthritis of the knee will end up with better mobility and, in most cases, less pain."

— *Tufts University Health & Nutrition Letter, October 1997*

"In an 18-month study, researchers at the Bowman Gray School of Medicine at Wake Forest University looked at the effect of exercise on 365 healthy people aged 60 and older who had osteoarthritis of the knee. Those who walked briskly or worked out with dumbbells and strap-on ankle weights for an hour three times a week were able to climb stairs, get out of cars, and perform other activities more easily and with less pain than the sedentary group."

— *Harvard Health Letter, March 1997*

These are just a few examples of the studies being conducted around the world that give evidence that exercise helps the symptoms of OA. But these results occur only with an *ongoing* and *regular* exercise program like the ACFP.

Exercise can improve—even relieve—the pain of osteoarthritis (OA). Exercise makes you more in tune with your body. By being a member of the Arthritis Cure Fitness Team you will be able to bet-

GETTING THE MOST OF THE CURE

The tremendous success of *The Arthritis Cure* had many positive consequences: millions of people felt relief from the painful symptoms of arthritis, and they were excited to be taking a proactive approach to managing their pain; supplement manufacturers saw tremendous growth in the demand for glucosamine and chondroitin; and people everywhere rejoiced that one of the most disabling diseases was finally easier to control.

Unfortunately, there were negative consequences too. Many of the dietary supplement manufacturers and marketers jumped on the bandwagon in an attempt to make a quick profit—but by marketing inferior versions of glucosamine and chondroitin. Consequently, people who were taking the inferior supplements were not realizing the full benefit of *The Arthritis Cure* program.

BUYER BEWARE: TIPS FOR CHOOSING A SUPPLEMENT

Because supplementation has recently become big business, there are many supplement companies that sell vast lines of products. Unfortunately, some of these companies even sell supplements that contain none of the active ingredients! For example, in a 1997 analysis of fifteen different brands of glucosamine and chondroitin supplements by the University of Maryland, researchers discovered that the amount found in the samples varied significantly from the amount printed on the label in many of the brands.

How does a concerned consumer make sure they're getting the true ingredients? Here are a few guidelines for being a smart supplement shopper.

1. STICK WITH A LARGE, REPUTABLE COMPANY. They have much more at stake than a small, unknown company. Rexall-Sundown, for example, is a company that enjoys a strong reputation in the supplement industry and is the only licensee of the patented glucosamine/chondroitin formula.

2. DON'T BE A BARGAIN SHOPPER. When it comes to nutritional supplements, buying the cheapest product isn't necessarily buying smart. Price should be but one factor that goes into your decision-making process.

3. PATENTS COUNT. A patent is a guarantee of quality for two reasons: First, since rigorous substantiation must be presented to the U.S. patent office before one is issued, you can be sure there is scientific research behind the product. Second, the product manufacturer must ensure that the product being sold contains the exact ingredients specified in the patent, or they will risk losing the patent. Dietary supplements that exist in nature—like chondroitin and glucosamine—are not patentable. The *combination* of glucosamine and chondroitin is patentable, so only buy a combined product if it clearly states "patented" on the label. For instance,

Osteo-Bi-Flex is a mass market brand of glucosamine and chondroitin that is authorized by the patent holder.

4. LOOK FOR THE WARNING LABEL. If a product makes a health claim, such as "helps maintain healthy, mobile joints and cartilage" then, by law, the manufacturer is required to run this statement: "These statements have not been evaluated by the Food and Drug Administration. This product is not intended to diagnose, treat, cure, or prevent any disease." If this wording isn't there, and the label makes such a health claim, then this company is running afoul of the law, and should be avoided. Who knows what other short cuts they may be taking?

5. CHECK THE PRODUCT EXPIRATION DATE. As supplements age, their potency diminishes, so keeping them around for too long is not a good idea. Remember if you buy large quantities, you may have supplements around for several months. Try to buy supplements with expiration dates *at least* nine months in the future.

ter determine the source of arthritic flare-ups, to differentiate between different types of "pain," to exercise at your own pace and according to your fitness level and degree of arthritis, and to know when it's OK—or not OK—to exercise. We will show you how to incorporate exercise for maximum results—relief from arthritis pain and a renewed sense of well-being.

Exercise is the key to managing osteoarthritis (glucosamine and chondroitin supplements help as well); however, "fitness" is not just physical. Fitness is personal—it is unique to you. It encompasses the physical, mental, emotional, and spiritual—either working in unison or at odds to make up the overall state of your well-being. Fitness includes how you feel about yourself, the world, your state of physical health, and what you do to take care of yourself.

For instance, you may be depressed that you have arthritis, and you may feel bitter that it has limited your activities. There will be days when you don't *feel* like exercising. On those days it is important not to let the emotional sabotage the physical. The Arthritis Cure Fitness Plan will not only strengthen you physically, but will lift your spirits and help you to better cope with arthritis.

Maybe you feel energized and ready to commit to an exercise program. It is important to start gradually and not to overdo it. Doing too much too soon may be discouraging if you expect results right away or if you experience excessive soreness from overworking your muscles. Through the Arthritis Cure Fitness Plan you will learn how to safely and effectively incorporate exercise into your life that will relieve painful joints and give you control over your disease.

Maybe you are overweight (as is the case with Barbara and many people with osteoarthritis) and for that reason have difficulty getting motivated to exercise. You know that exercising will help take the weight off but those excess pounds make it all the more difficult. The Arthritis Cure Fitness Plan will help you get over that "hump." Soon those pounds will be coming off and exercise will, like sleeping or eating, become a natural part of your life.

When considering your overall fitness it is important to think about your relationship with food. A healthy diet and exercise go together. If you begin the Arthritis Cure Fitness Plan but continue bad eating habits, such as eating fast foods, fried foods or processed foods, you may not get the results you expect. We will give you a plan for healthy eating and balanced nutrition that will promote weight loss and make you feel great—even with arthritis!

If you are familiar with *The Arthritis Cure* you already know about the benefits of taking glucosamine and chondroitin supplements. Millions of people have experienced noticeable, positive results after taking these natural arthritis pain alleviators. Glucosamine and chondroitin supplements, as recommended in *The Arthritis Cure*, should be incorporated into your overall fitness plan for alleviating your arthritis. However, if you haven't read *The Arthritis Cure* and you haven't yet tried glucosamine and chondroitin, you can still benefit from the information in this book.

Regular exercise, improved eating habits and supplements, along with a new awareness of how your mind and body play out a magnificent symphony (you are the conductor) will make a significant difference in how you view and live your life. Yet, the attrition rate of people—especially older people—with arthritis who begin an exercise program is high. In one study, nearly half of the older people had stopped exercising eighteen months after beginning. Most studies of middle-aged and older people suggest only a 50 percent adherence rate by twelve to twenty-four months after initiating an exercise program.[2]

Do the best thing you could possibly do for yourself: don't be one of the 50 percent that stops forever. Be like Barbara and find a way to get exercise back into your life, and make it a permanent part of your life. Try to envision yourself a year from now. What do you see? Do you see progress? You have good reason to. You have all the tools you need to become that happy, healthy, and active person you envision. Let's get started!

CHAPTER TWO

Pain 101

*Dealing with stress is a daily challenge. By learning to man-
age your stress in a positive way, you can reduce your pain, feel
healthier and manage your disease more effectively.*

—ARTHRITIS FOUNDATION, "MANAGING YOUR STRESS"

YOU MAY ALREADY KNOW A GOOD DEAL about the mechan-
ics of OA, or at least you've *experienced* the mechanics first-hand. But
the more you know about your disease, the more you can do to help
yourself, and the sooner the healing process will begin.

OSTEOARTHRITIS: WHAT IT IS

Osteoarthritis is the most common type of arthritis. It generally
afflicts weight-bearing joints like knees or hips, although OA in
finger joints occurs in approximately 70 percent of people over age
sixty-five.[1] It can also occur in the large joint at the base of the big
toe, or in the spine creating stiffness and pain in the neck, base of
head, legs, lower back, and arms. OA in the knee accounts for as
much disability in older Americans as diabetes, heart disease, hip
fractures, and depression.[2] Studies show that 5 percent of people
who leave the workforce do so because of the limitations imposed by
OA. That's second only to problems caused by heart disease.[3] It's
estimated that by the year 2020, about sixty million people will
experience the pain caused by this condition.[4]

OA is typically associated with people who are obese because the
excess weight the joints have to manage wears away cartilage. The
fact is, middle-aged women who are overweight can reduce their
chances of acquiring OA simply by losing weight. The Arthritis

DON'T GO IT ALONE

Jan, a 68-year-old, overweight woman goes to her doctor complaining of pain in her knees. The pain occurs primarily when she walks, but gets worse when she goes up and down stairs. She often fears that her knee will "give out." One knee swells on occasion. When she wakes up in the morning, or after a period of inactivity, she experiences between ten and fifteen minutes of stiffness in her knees, and sometimes in her hands. Her doctor tells her it's osteoarthritis, and suggests she take acetaminophen or ibuprofen.[18]

She does. It provides some relief. But things don't get better. She feels depressed, unmotivated, and reluctant to exercise because it hurts, and the extra weight she carries makes it unpleasant. Her physical condition worsens, and soon, she's taking nonsteroidal anti-inflammatory drugs (NSAIDs) like Naproxen. They help the pain, but she's leery of the side effects. Her depression deepens. She doesn't feel like seeing anyone. She's starting to feel angry. Her body hurts. Her heart aches. She may eat for comfort, or not eat at all. Life has lost its spark.

Many experiences with arthritis begin like Jan's. A physician checks the range of motion, tenderness, and pain when bending or flexing the joint. A diagnosis is made, and some recommendations for how to deal with it are given. But it's what happens *after* the patient leaves the doctor's office that determines how well he or she will *cope* with the pain, depression, and diminished quality of life associated with OA.

Like Jan, some people try to "go it alone." Unfortunately, many end up *feeling* alone. But research shows that those who learn about their condition—and find support groups or people with whom they can share their feelings—not only know they're not alone, but they may even experience less physical distress.

The conclusions of one recent study showed that patients who had arthritis who participated in a program to self-manage their pain and rehabilitation experienced a substantial decline in pain and depression, as well as a reduced need for the use of health services—this despite a 9 percent increase in their physical disability. The study also showed that the more patients knew about their condition, the more confidence they felt in their ability to cope both physically and emotionally.[19] Dr. Kate Lorig, associate professor of research at Stanford University Medical Center and director of Stanford's Patient Education Resource Center, conducted the study and reports, "Like all paths, there are ups and there are downs, but having the skills to deal with the downs make continuing on the path a lot easier." Dr. Lorig says that after four years of participating in a self-care program, patients had 20 percent less pain and 40 percent fewer doctors' visits than patients who had never taken a self-management program. Lorig says that the self-help programs are of value to people in many ways, from overcoming their fear of falling, to finding ways to realize lifelong dreams. The most effective programs are those that deal directly with pain management.[20]

Foundation claims that women who lose eleven pounds over a ten year period can reduce their risk of OA by 50 percent![5]

More men are diagnosed with OA prior to age forty-five. After age fifty-four, however, it is twice as common in women than in men. In America, OA in the hips is fairly common, and men outnumber women with afflictions of the hip. They tend to feel pain around their groin, inner thigh, buttocks and outside thigh. It may feel worse when they walk (although we'll explain why it's important to keep walking anyway).

Women experience the condition more in their hands and knees[6] and it is genetically more likely to occur in the knees of black women than in white women. Those with OA in the knees (equaling about 14 percent of all who suffer from OA)[7] may experience a grating, catching feeling that worsens when they go up or down stairs or get up or down from sitting in a chair.

When OA is present in the fingers, it may manifest as nodules at the upper joints, called Heberden's nodes, or nodes in the lower finger joints known as Bouchard's nodes. Heberden nodes can appear on women as young as forty, and tend to follow a genetic predisposition. Even though those with OA in their fingers will generally still have good use of their hands, they might regularly experience a tingling or numbing in the fingers.

It's common that individuals with OA feel pain in only one knee, elbow, hip, or finger even though those same joints on the opposite side of the body may show cartilage deterioration in an X ray. In fact, curiously enough, OA is often present within a joint, even though the individual may feel no pain whatsoever. Research shows that only one-third of identifiable cases actually cause pain.[8] But, most experts agree there are approximately sixteen million Americans who *do* feel the pain.

For those who do feel pain, they say that it comes and goes and symptoms usually start off slowly and may not seem significant at first. Pain occurs more in the evening hours than the morning, and many people believe humidity makes the pain worse (some claim it helps). Stiffness might be worse after periods of overuse or inactivity, such as after sleeping or sitting down for long periods of time. People who choose not to exercise or move their affected joints at all will generally become weaker and the pain will become more intense. That's because weak muscles cannot efficiently support joints, which results, again, in more pain.[9]

THE OVERWHELMING EMOTIONAL IMPACT

Aside from physical disability, few people are prepared for the emotional impact OA imposes on their lives.

Chronic pain and stiffness in the knees doesn't just limit your ability to go up or down stairs; it can restrict every movement and activity, and impact your overall lifestyle.

OA may be centered in your joints, but its impact spreads to work lives as well as home lives. It can keep you from participating in athletic activities, prevent you from enjoying social events, and even impede the most simple enjoyments of life like playing with your grandchildren. For some, it even tarnishes their spiritual or religious beliefs or causes depression.

When you're depressed, you may avoid straining yourself with physical exertion. In turn, your muscles weaken and joints begin to atrophy. In fact, joints that are immobilized for as short a time as four months can begin a series of changes that result in significant destruction of the entire joint (even in the *absence* of disease). The deteriorating physical condition is a vicious cycle leading to more depression, which leads to less mobility, weaker muscles, malnourished joints, more depression, and so on.

GAINING ALTITUDE

It is important to look at the bigger picture. If you can see your emotional ups and downs as a symptom of the disease rather than as yet another "disease," then you may be able to address your condition with more reason, hope, and positive results. This includes taking command of your recuperation by exercising; finding ways to cope with the depression by making new social contacts possibly through support groups; eating well; and taking the appropriate medications and supplements when necessary.[21] Creating your own fitness program based on the Arthritis Cure Fitness Plan will boost your energy level and confidence. It's ultimately up to you to commit to an overall fitness program.

Healthy Joints and Cartilage Matrix

Osteoarthritis is also known as degenerative joint disease. That's because cartilage within the joint deteriorates, leaving the bones they were once protecting exposed and rubbing up against each other. The function of a joint is to provide flexibility, support, stability, and protection.[10] It does that successfully when water, collagen, proteoglycans, and substances called chondrocytes make up what is known as a healthy "cartilage matrix."

Joints are made up of a great deal of cartilage, which is a firm, rubbery substance that blankets the ends of our bones. Cartilage is slicker than ice, and enables our joints to glide smoothly between the motions of our bones. Due to its sponge-like nature, cartilage also acts as a sophisticated shock absorber, so when we run, jump, bump or just get jolted somehow, our bones don't collide. Essentially, cartilage softens the blows, making us resilient. So, even though we may not like the bumps, jolts, and jumps, we are at least walking away, most of the time, without injury.[11]

If we take a closer look at a healthy joint, we see lots of fluid. Cartilage is made up mostly of water; between 65 and 80 percent of it. A substance called synovial fluid provides the cartilage with nourishment (cartilage is one of very few of our body parts that doesn't have a direct link to blood, which nourishes the rest of our body). So, having enough synovial fluid is crucial for healthy cartilage.

When a joint is resting, the cartilage is filled with synovial fluid. But when there's pressure against the joint, the fluid is squeezed out of the spongy cartilage. This is the normal, healthy job of the cartilage, and absorbing and expelling of the fluid is what keeps things circulating around the joints.

Collagen is important for a properly functioning joint because it gives the joint its elasticity while also holding together the entire cartilage matrix. Both collagen and proteoglycans (a substance that weaves through the collagen, enabling it to "bounce back" when it's stretched or restricted) are made from chondrocytes. But chondrocytes also produce enzymes that destroy collagen and proteoglycans that have become old and are no longer useful.

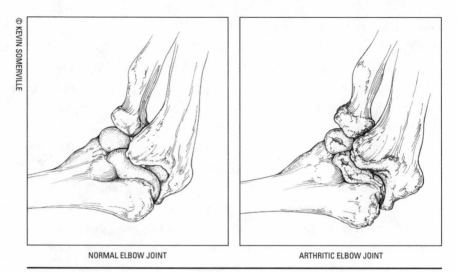

NORMAL ELBOW JOINT | ARTHRITIC ELBOW JOINT

Wearing Thin

If we look closely at a joint affected by osteoarthritis, we see that the cartilage is thin, pitted, or broken down and has lost its ability to protect opposing bones from grinding against each other, causing agonizing pain or stiffness. There may be a loss of synovial fluid, the cartilage dries out, loses its elasticity, and no longer performs as a shock absorber; it also causes pain. Subsequently, the cartilage cracks, creating bone spurs (or osteophytes). The bones themselves can harden causing a condition known as eburnation. Or, the bone might harbor fluid-filled pockets called subchondral cysts. There may also be tiny bits of broken bones lodging themselves in the joint like sharp needles.

In some cases, the cartilage mix has gone awry, and the chondrocytes release enzymes that do away with the good collagen and proteoglycans as well as the bad. That can cause a build up of synovial fluid that then washes away the productive chemicals that keep the joint healthy. Alternatively, it may flood the joint cavity, creating pain and swelling.

Meanwhile, the condition progresses and the bare bones continue to rub up against each other, until, with time, the condition can cause deformities, inflammation, stiffness, and pain.

Primary and Secondary OA

There are two kinds of OA: primary and secondary. Primary is more common, and comes on slowly and progressively. It generally hits people over the age of forty-five, and seems to manifest either after:

- excessive weight is applied to regular joints over and over again, or
- when reasonable weight is applied to inferior joints.

Obesity is the perfect breeding ground for primary OA since excessive weight constantly forces itself upon joints designed to operate under much less stress. But genetics play their role, too. It's estimated that approximately six million people inherit OA through their family tree.[12]

Secondary arthritis is generally caused by a trauma, injury, or

AGE DOES NOT EQUAL OA!

Contrary to what medical doctors have believed for generations, turning sixty does not absolutely mean that your knees will start to ache, and your elbows start to creak. We now know that OA is not a normal, inevitable part of aging. Aging *does* take it's toll, but it's easy to identify OA—if you know what you're looking for:

1. Age affects the health of *non-weight bearing* joints, while osteoarthritis attacks *weight-bearing* joints.

2. Age-worn joints don't display any chemical changes within the cartilage, but the cartilage in people with OA undergoes a chemical change—there is no pigment in the cartilage, and it might be either dried up or unnecessarily filled with fluid.

3. Normal "older" joint tissues don't increase in volume, nor do their bones change. People with OA, however, will have increased tissue volume and a change in their bones.

So, if you have OA, it means you have experienced a chemical change within your body. And exercising regularly is *not* responsible for that chemical change. On the contrary, we now know that regular exercise increases the function of people who have primary OA, and it can *prevent* primary OA in those who start out with the secondary kind.[22]

infection, and often occurs in people before they reach the age of forty. But the joint itself doesn't necessarily have to be injured to cause the deterioration. Rather, for example, a sports injury tearing a ligament may create enough trauma on the joint so that it eventually wears down. People who play football or soccer are at higher risk for OA, as are those whose jobs require constant knee-bending activities.[13] "Trick knees," calcium deposits, and constant repetitive actions like pitching a baseball, lifting heavy boxes, or ballet dancing all play into the manifestation of secondary arthritis.[14]

Osteoarthritis: What It Is Not

Although OA is the most common type of arthritis, it shouldn't be lumped together or confused with either *rheumatoid arthritis* or *osteoporosis*, as these are three very different conditions.

Rheumatoid arthritis (RA) is an immune-system disorder in which the antibodies within the body attack the joint as if it was invading the body. Consequently, the joints become red and inflamed. As it progresses, it can lead to weakness, fatigue, fever, anemia, and other profoundly difficult or painful conditions.

Unlike OA, where one knee or one elbow might be affected while the other is not, the nature of RA is that it tends to affect the body symmetrically. In other words, both knees, both elbows, or both wrists tend to be affected. In this type of arthritis, the cartilage and bones within a joint do not deteriorate.

ATTENTION ALL MEN

Feel like it's too late to get started with a workout program? Here's news for you men out there who think couch potato status is just fine: Studies show that men between 45 to 84 years of age who take up brisk walking, swimming, or other moderately vigorous activities have a 23 to 29 percent lower death rate than non-exercisers. On top of that, they reduce their chances of getting heart disease by 14 percent. Even those men who wait until they retire, or age 65, to begin working out, gain life expectancy.

RA is generally treated quite differently than OA. (For more information on the cause, physics, and how to treat RA see "The Arthritis Foundation" in *Resources*).

Unlike either OA or RA, *osteoporosis* is a condition in which bone mass deteriorates. Again, cartilage is unaffected. Since the reconstructive mechanisms of bones slow down after age thirty-five, people who don't supplement their diets with bone-building supplements such as calcium and vitamin D may experience the affects of osteoporosis. This is especially common in post-menopausal women.

The following chart compares and contrasts many aspects of OA, RA, and osteoporosis.[15]

Osteoarthritis	Rheumatoid Arthritis	Osteoporosis
Begins after age 40	Strikes between 25-50	Occurs late in life
Develops gradually	Comes and goes without warning	Gradual onslaught
Hits single joints	Attacks joints on both sides of body	Affects bone mass
Inflammation atypical	Inflammation universal	No inflammation
Affects weight-bearing joints	Affects all joints	Affects bone mass
Isolated pain	Pain, fatigue all over	Usually painless
Exercise Helps	Exercise might help	Exercise may prevent
Diet helps	Diet may help	Diet can prevent

MEDICAL BAND-AIDS

Doctors used to believe that OA was incurable. Indeed, in many books or reference materials circulating around these days, it's still labeled as incurable. Historically, that's why prescription drugs were chosen for the majority of cases. The objective of both the doctor and patient was to relieve the pain. If they succeeded, they thought they were doing all that could be done.

But the potent nonsteroidal anti-inflammatory drugs (NSAIDs) most commonly used have a down side. Each year thousands of people die from the side-effects of these products. Furthermore, masking pain with drugs doesn't address the root of the problem, nor does it help rehabilitate the condition.

Many people who take NSAIDs and avoid exercise eventually face what they think is inevitable: surgery. But there is no guarantee the surgery will work, it's expensive, and it can also be very difficult, especially for the elderly, to recover completely.

The best news for people these days is that exercise, the use of glucosamine and chondroitin, and diet can make an enormous difference in both alleviating pain and keeping the joint as healthy as possible.[16]

EXERCISE AND OSTEOARTHRITIS: A GOOD RELATIONSHIP

Whether the cause of osteoarthritis is primary and genetic, or secondary and can be targeted to an old injury, research shows that strengthening the muscles that surround the affected joint is a very effective therapy. Stronger muscles not only work for the joint by acting as a substitute shock absorber, but exercise, as it is strengthening muscle, also requires more synovial fluid to enter the remaining cartilage. That means more oxygen and nutrients are delivered to the "sick" cartilage. In short, the more nutrients the cartilage receives, the more likely it is to maintain or regain its health.[17]

CHAPTER THREE

The Mechanics of Exercise

"If exercise could be packed into a pill, it would be the single most widely prescribed and beneficial medicine in the nation."

—NATIONAL INSTITUTE ON AGING

WHY DOES REGULAR EXERCISE help people manage the pain they experience with OA?

When we do something as simple as lift a grocery bag, or as strenuous as running a marathon, we are essentially asking our bodies to produce more energy. And as part of that requirement, our muscles, nervous, cardiovascular, and respiratory systems, as well as our bones are put to work and asked to produce. The substances they produce, such as oxygen, carbon dioxide, calcium, and nutrients, are of great benefit to our bodily systems. Plus, the energy that's produced helps eliminate toxins or other invaders from our bodies, keeping our systems cleaner and running more efficiently.

Some exercises and activities use more muscles than others do, just as some exercises require more stamina than others. But our bodies are like machines in that each organ, muscle, ligament, tendon, joint, limb, and even our flesh is affected by the use of any of the other parts.

BENEFITS OF EXERCISE:

1. Improves cardiovascular system.
2. Helps control weight.
3. Builds muscles.
4. Improves blood fat and reduces cholesterol.
5. Boosts glucose (sugar) metabolism.
6. Lowers blood pressure.
7. Maintains or increases bone density.
8. Improves state of mind.
9. Slows aging process.
10. Relieves pain from osteoarthritis.

If you don't use and keep the muscles in your body toned, they will eventually lose their ability to contract, or to support those body parts they are responsible for holding together. The result is structural damage to other parts of the body like ligaments, bones, or joints. For example, if you have pain in one of your knees when you walk, you may shift your weight to relieve the pressure on the knee that hurts. The consequence of that, however, may be that over time the hip on which the bulk of your weight is placed may become strained and may itself become arthritic.

Through exercise you can strengthen the muscles around your afflicted knee. As you strengthen the muscles that support your knee, they will not only act as a better shock absorber, thereby relieving some of the pain, but they will also—without painful consequence—take the weight off your knee joint and carry the weight that was intended for your knee.

THE JOINT EFFORT

Joints are made to move. Their entire design tells us that. For example, when a knee joint is relaxed (in a sitting position with no pressure on the joint), the cartilage within the joints are expanded and filled with the nutritional synovial fluid. This is good for your joint since the fluid provides it with essential nutrients.

When the joint has pressure on it (standing position), the synovial fluid is squeezed out of the cartilage and the expelling of old fluid makes way for the importing of new, more nutritious fluid.

HANDS-ON HEALING!

While constructing your program for optimum health, consider getting a regular massage. Not only is it relaxing and rejuvenating, but it also invigorates muscles, tendons, and ligaments. For those who get caught up in the demands of everyday life, massage may be the only time you can completely relax, contemplate, and be nurtured. Massage also helps relieve anxiety and depression, and makes you more aware of your body and what it needs to be healthy. Massage is an investment in yourself.

When OA is present in the knee joint, sitting or being inactive for long periods of time creates an excess build-up of fluid, creating stiffness and pain when the joint is finally moved. Standing for long periods, on the other hand, doesn't allow for the joint to soak up new nutritious fluid, which can also cause pain. Consequently if you remain sedentary your arthritic knee will become immobile.

When you don't challenge your muscles through exercise, your joint can also become hypermobile. Hypermobility is a result of loose ligaments that no longer work well with the joint. The joint becomes "floppy" and the muscles surrounding the joint turn sore as they try to compensate for the looseness of the joint and ligament. So to avoid joint immobility *or* hypermobility the key is to get moving with the Arthritis Cure Fitness Plan!

THE LEGACY OF EXERCISE

For people who suffer from OA, regular exercise is beneficial for many different reasons. It can help you have a better sense of control, improve balance, provide a better quality of sleep, elevate reaction time, help regulate breathing patterns and internal body

EXERCISE AND OSTEOARTHRITIS

Exercise is critical to health of osteoarthritic joints because it:

• strengthens muscles so they are more able to protect joints by absorbing shock.
• improves stability.
• helps joint flexibility, lessening pain and decreasing the risk of sprains and other injuries.
• stops the progression of osteoarthritis.

On the other hand lack of exercise may cause:

• weakened and inflexible muscles, tendons, and ligaments.
• cartilage in an arthritic joint to thin and soften, making it unable to perform its buffering job.
• pieces of bone to break off and lodge into nerves.
• joints to become "fixed" and immobile.
• withdrawal and depression.

temperature, and boost self-esteem. Exercise can also reduce the risk of:

- heart disease
- adult-onset diabetes
- colon cancer
- breast cancer
- prostate cancer
- falling and subsequent fractures
- high blood pressure
- obesity
- depression
- osteoporosis
- frailty resulting from age

For generations, the common belief about exercise and OA was that vigorous activity over time actually *caused* the joint stress that contributed to the cartilage breakdown. Try to erase everything you've ever heard about how exercise is bad for OA. Experts across the board now agree that exercise is crucial.

PHYSICAL FITNESS AND OA

The Arthritis Cure Fitness Plan includes four areas of physical fitness that, if applied, will improve your condition. They are:

1. strength
2. aerobic capacity
3. flexibility
4. agility/balance

Strength

The best reason to begin the Arthritis Cure Fitness Plan is to strengthen your muscles. Strong muscles surrounding an arthritic joint relieve the joint of carrying too much weight and act as joint

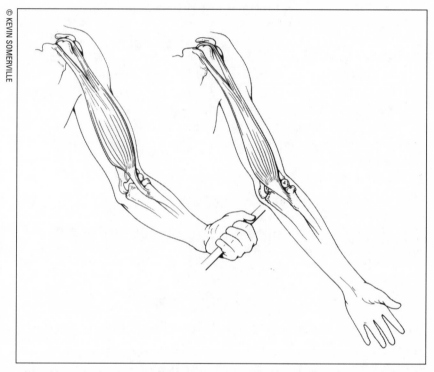

A healthy, exercised muscle (left) next to an unchallenged, atrophied muscle (right).

shock absorbers. The result is less pain. Strengthening muscles also increases bone mass, which has prophylactic effects on arthritis.

A strong muscle is defined by its capacity to exert force through the contractions of muscle fibers. The size of a muscle determines its strength, but don't worry, you don't have to be a muscle-bound bodybuilder to participate in the Arthritis Cure Fitness Plan (and it won't turn you into one). The Arthritis Cure Fitness Plan *will* challenge and strengthen the muscles you have regardless of size, and improve muscle endurance.[1]

GETTING A JUMP ON MOBILITY AND EXERCISE

What types of exercise are best for people with OA?

Most people perceive exercise to mean more than doing household chores or walking to the end of the frontwalk to pick up the newspaper. If, however, you experience terrible pain when you walk, bend, or reach, those activities may seem like plenty. And to begin with, they may be.

But there are choices you can make within the framework of your day that will provide you with a few more opportunities to be more active. For instance, you can park at the far end of a parking lot and walk to a store, rather than parking close in. Maybe you can mow the lawn yourself instead of hiring the teenager next door to do it. All these seemingly small choices contribute to a much larger picture of health. Whatever you choose to do remember to do it at your own pace—listen to your body—but don't "sit still" for your disease to progress unnecessarily.

No matter how insignificant the changes may seem, now is a good time to start recognizing when and how you can make those extra efforts. They will signal to your brain that you are gearing up for the Arthritis Cure Fitness Plan— even if that means easing into it one small step at a time. Sometimes you may take two steps forward and take one step back. But stick to it. Resolve to make more mobility, more activity, more open-minded choices about how to construct a healthier day.

Endurance is the ability of muscles to *repeat* contractions against resistance over a specific period of time. It is also measured by the amount of time you can *sustain* a specific muscle contraction. The more you demand of your muscles to repeat and sustain contractions, the more they will be able to repeat and sustain contractions. In other words, the more you demand of your muscles, the more they'll produce. Meanwhile, the more you demand, the more you stimulate increased blood flow, which in turn, feeds oxygen, nutrients, and enzymes to the muscle, warding off fatigue.[2]

Lifting free weights or using muscle-strengthening machines are typically how strengthening and improving endurance occurs most efficiently. But if you're not ready for this level, the force of gravity can provide enough resistance and you can do muscle strengthening exercises without using weights. The Arthritis Cure Fitness Plan includes muscle strengthening exercises for all the major muscle groups and can be done with or without weights and according to your level of fitness.

Aerobic Capacity

Your ability to keep moving (stamina) while working your muscles is how aerobic capacity is measured. Generally speaking, if the activity you're participating in boosts your heart rate for between fifteen and twenty minutes, you are engaged in aerobic exercise.

Running, walking, swimming, biking, dancing, rowing—all these activities and many more test or build your aerobic capacity. They also promote healthier bones that can act as shock absorbers for ineffective joints, and shed pounds that may be stressing the joints. Water aerobics is a most beneficial type of aerobic activity for people with osteoarthritis.

Aerobic exercise is defined as any type of physical conditioning performed to increase respiration and heart rate. When you swim,

BUILDING MUSCLE STRENGTH AND ENDURANCE

There are three basic methods to improve strength and endurance of a muscle:

1. ISOMETRIC FORCE: contracting a muscle and holding it still for several seconds. For instance, lifting a weight and holding it in the air straight in front of you for six seconds. Isometric activities work only on isolated muscles and don't provide a good overall strengthening and endurance program.

2. DYNAMIC OR ISOTONIC FORCE: contracting a muscle and moving it through its range of motion. For instance, a biceps curl: holding a weight with your hand at your side, then flexing the elbow, bringing the weight to your shoulder and back down again. Free weights or weight-bearing exercise machines at gyms provide this kind of strengthening. The more these are done, the more resistance you'll be able to lift and move. This type of movement also creates motion with joints. This is excellent for overall toning, especially if you do these types of moves on several different muscles.

3. ISOKINETIC FORCE: speed of the contraction remains constant, but resistance from the machine (usually required for this type of contraction) matches the individual's level of strength throughout the range of motion. This type of conditioning is more complicated and is usually done at the gym with a certified professional trainer or physical therapist.

THE BASICS OF STRETCHING

There are three types of stretching of which you should be aware:

1. STATIC STRETCHES: Moving the joint to lengthen the muscle and tendons, holding the stretch for between 20 and 30 seconds. For example, push the fingers of one hand down with the palm of the other hand until you feel the wrist muscles and tendons stretch. Static stretches are safe, as long as you don't push to the point of pain. Over time, these stretches will increase mobility and flexibility.

2. BALLISTIC STRETCHES: A dangerous kind of stretching involving bouncing or jerking of the muscles and tendons. You may see runners using ballistic stretches as they bend over and reach for their toes. Their stretches often bounce at the waist. This is not recommended, however, since it can result in injury.

3. DYNAMIC STRETCHES: There is no bouncing or jerking; rather, the joint's full range-of-motion is checked while the tendons and muscles are stretched. Refer back to the static stretch of your wrist. You could take that stretch one step farther by moving your wrist in slow, careful circles while it is in its most stretched position.

for example, your heart is pumping blood to the muscles you're working. And the more efficiently your heart is delivering the goods, the longer you'll be able to swim continuously.

Your heart isn't the only organ at work during aerobic activity; your lungs, arteries, capillaries, cells, and veins all contribute to carrying the oxygen, carbon dioxide, and other nutrients to the muscle. They also help eliminate wastes from the muscles. Meanwhile, the muscles you're working rely on glycogen for fuel, which is conveniently stored within the muscles themselves. As long as there's enough fuel and oxygenated blood being sent to the working muscles, you won't feel fatigued. If, however, you exercise beyond the capacity of your muscles to feed off the nutrients, then lactic acid builds up within the muscle, and causes fatigue. That's the point at which you feel like you can no longer go on, and exclaim, "Enough!"

You can build up your aerobic endurance and create a change in your physiological structure through four different means. You can remember it by recommitting yourself to your goal and getting fit, but in this case, FITT:

- Frequency: the more often you do it, the more quickly changes will occur.
- Intensity: the more intense your workout, the sooner the changes will occur.

- Time: the longer you engage in the aerobics, the greater impact it will have on your body.
- Type of exercise: If you swim, you'll demand change in different muscles than if you ride a bike. Cross training, which we'll talk about later, is a good idea since it ultimately covers most of the muscle groups within your body.

The types of physiological changes you can expect include favorable improvements with:

REST IS ESSENTIAL

Working out isn't all you need for improved health. Rest is important, too. In addition to resting the affected joints between training sessions, it's crucial to take a break when a joint becomes painful during exercise. When the knee or elbow is affected, a neoprene or elastic brace or taping may help stabilize the joint during exercise and reduce pain. Any activity that causes pain lasting for more than two hours should not be repeated.[3]

- Resting heart rate and blood pressure, submaximal exercise heart rate, and blood pressure and body weight
- Body composition (the percentages of the body that are muscle and bone by comparison to body fat)
- Lipoproteins (chemical structures present in the blood that carry fat, proteins, and cholesterol)
- Fat and carbohydrate metabolism (the way the body uses fat and sugar carried in the blood)
- Bone mineralization

(Regular aerobic workouts do all that *and* make you feel better emotionally!)

Flexibility

Most people with OA have limited flexibility and range-of-motion in the affected joints. And due to the inflexibility, it's easy to strain or sprain the adjoining muscles, and stress out other parts of the body that are trying to compensate for the static areas. This is why it is *so* important to regain flexibility in the places that are slowly becoming immobile.

Keeping a joint flexible will prevent injury. Flexible joints also enhance the ability for muscles to become stronger because muscles can operate through their full range of motion without limitations. Stretching is the best way to improve flexibility, and regardless of your condition, you can start a stretching program *today* with the Arthritis Cure Fitness Plan.

Stretching requires no equipment, no fees, nobody else, and can be done just about anywhere.

Yoga is an excellent vehicle for good stretching and enhancing flexibility, and can be practiced by anyone. Massage, dancing, martial arts, and water aerobics are just a few other ways to improve flexibility.

Agility/Balance

Measuring agility and balance is slightly more elusive than measuring the other types of fitness. Some people are more coordinated in one activity than another. Standing on one foot may be difficult for you, but chasing after tennis balls might be a cinch.

The important thing to remember here is that maintaining balance and agility is vital for your overall well-being. By designing an exercise program in which you cross train, you can pretty much be guaranteed that your agility and balance will increase. Dance, martial arts, yoga, tennis, even badminton are all activities that engender greater coordination. Improving agility and balance is especially important for arthritis sufferers because it: 1) makes you more active, 2) helps give your joints and muscles better range of motion, 3) increases your flexibility, and 4) boosts your overall confidence.

Aging has far less to do with the loss of strength, flexibility, agility, and cardiovascular capabilities than does immobility. All types of fitness are lost at the same rate when we slow our activities, or avoid exercise altogether. For instance, if you lose flexibility, you will automatically lose some agility, strength, and cardiovascular ability. Likewise, if you improve your strength, you'll automatically inspire better flexibility. If you work out aerobically, you'll also enable better balance. Remember, your body is a complex machine, and each part is dependent on another. Start a good ripple effect by getting yourself going through exercise—it's within *your* control.

CHAPTER FOUR

The Right Way to a Good Exercise Program

"If you believe you can, or if you believe you cannot, you will be right."

—HENRY FORD

SHOULD I ALWAYS WARM UP before exercise? How should I warm up? Is cooling down as important as warming up? When should I inhale and exhale? Is "no pain, no gain" the universal axiom for getting the most out of exercise?

These are common questions for anyone beginning an exercise program. Even seasoned athletes need to keep up with the latest, most efficient, and safest ways to achieve fitness, which can change on a monthly basis.

The best news about adhering to the Arthritis Cure Fitness Plan is that it will make your exercise routine enjoyable, effective, and easy. You *can* exercise safely and effectively—even with arthritis—by doing the following:

1. **Consult your physician.** This is important for *anyone* starting a fitness program but *crucial* for osteoarthritis sufferers. Everyone's body is different. Your doctor should assess how advanced your arthritis is and the level of exercise you can endure. This will help you design your own fitness plan.

2. **Reaffirm Your Goals.** Make a list of goals that you would like to achieve through the Arthritis Cure Fitness Plan. Read them each day before you exercise. Adjust your goals if, as you are exercising, they seem too unrealistic or too simplistic. Many athletes use visualization

to improve their performance before a sporting event. Whatever you do, start each routine by affirming that you are going to stick to the program.

3. Wear Appropriate Clothing. Often an excuse *not* to exercise is physical discomfort from inappropriate clothing. The proper attire for your workout may make a world of difference! If it's hot where you're walking, wear light, breathable fabrics like cotton; if you're setting out for a cross country ski, take appropriate layers of clothing so you can bundle up if the wind whips up, or peel off if the sun gets too hot.

4. Choose Activities You Enjoy. It may take some experimenting, but there are many options when it comes to exercise. It is

THESE SHOES WERE MADE FOR WALKING

Everyone who exercises needs a pair of comfortable shoes to match the needs of their feet and the type of exercise they are doing. It's easy to figure out what kind of shoes to use: simply ask yourself what you're going to be doing—shoes are made with a specific activity in mind. If walking is your exercise of choice, get a walking shoe—they have more flexibility in the instep. If you plan on plenty of tennis, get a good tennis or court shoe—they are made to help you with the lateral action and quick stops and starts. If you're going to take aerobics, buy an aerobics shoe—they are cushioned to absorb the impact to the knees, ankles, and feet. And it makes sense to have several different pairs of shoes if you're going to engage in several different kinds of exercise.

For those with low arches, try inserting a custom-made foot orthotic that can reestablish a normal arch. By the way, you may find that you wear a larger size in sporting shoes than in street shoes.

People with high arches should get shoes with very cushioned midsoles and a deep toe area—the toe area needs to accommodate the increased thickness at the ball of the foot.

Whatever you do, shop around and ask questions. People who really know the shoe business will be able to answer your questions and guide you to the perfect fit. Don't be hasty, though. Buying and using good shoes may be one of the most important steps you can take to avoid injuries and successfully reach your fitness goals.

important, however, not to force yourself to participate in an exercise that you simply don't like. There's no reason to swim if you can't bear to get wet!

5. Find Comfortable Conditions. Each type of exercise has its disadvantages. Be honest with yourself about what they are and how they might impact you. Your commitment is key. Don't let the little things bring you down. If you take up swimming, be sure the temperature at the pool you visit will remain constant, and make sure the hours match your schedule. Before you buy a bike, make sure traffic, rain, and an occasional flat tire don't bother you. If aerobics classes interest you, take time to interview the instructor, explaining your special needs to be sure you're in the right hands.

6. Use Safety Gear. Don't hesitate to use devices that might help you exercise with arthritis—for example, a kickboard, innertube, or rubber shoes while swimming. Don't neglect the usual safety guidelines like wearing a helmet when bicycling or knee, wrist, and elbow guards when rollerblading.

7. Determine What, How Often, and When. Look carefully at your habits, your schedule, and the

EVERY MOVE YOU MAKE

Whether you're standing, sitting, laying down, or doing the watusi, how you hold yourself, or your posture, plays a big part in maintaining good health.

If you're on your feet for long hours, be sure to invest in the proper shoes (use a high stool to sit in, if possible). Rotate your weight so you don't spend much more time on one side or the other. Try keeping your knees "loose" when you stand squarely over your feet. Stand tall and erect with your shoulders high, not rounded. If you have trouble with your back or posture, consult a chiropractor or other health care practitioner for tips on how to adjust.

If you sit a lot, working at a desk or computer, for instance, invest in a chair that provides good back support. Make sure it's easy for you to sit down into it, and then to get up out of it.

When you sleep, don't lie on your stomach if you can help it. If you can't help it, place a pillow under your pelvis. If you sleep on your side, place a pillow between your knees. When on your back, place a pillow under your knees. Make sure your mattress is comfortable and suits your needs.

Posture in every position can help with the dynamics of a stronger, happier body.

ATHLETE'S FOOT

If you are one of the many people who suffer from athlete's foot, don't worry. Exercise won't make it worse if you:

• Wear only cotton socks.
• Change your socks several times a day.
• Dry your feet thoroughly after bathing.
• Wear shoes that "breathe," allowing air to circulate through the shoe.

demands your routine places on you (i.e., you may want to walk while it's still light outside or you may have more energy in the morning) and commit to the times of day you will exercise. That can change daily if necessary, but allotting time to exercise will help you avoid distractions and stick to the program.

8. **Get professional instruction.** Whether you decide to work out with free weights or machines, ride a bike, swim—even walk—it would be wise to get a few hours of advice from a professional trainer. We will show you the elements of the Arthritis Cure Fitness Plan, but you may want a professional to help you with the application.

9. **Cross Train.** Cross training keeps your muscles toned evenly, preventing biochemical or structural imbalances in your body. It also keeps you from being bored with the same exercises. If you walk twice a week, ride a bike twice a week, and work out on weights twice a week, you'll not only look and feel better, you'll also be more inclined to stick with it because it won't become tedious.

10. **Be Consistent.** It is *essential* that you be consistent. You could set yourself up for injury if you exercise only every now and then, and you won't gain positive results from the Arthritis Cure Fitness Plan if you do it sporadically.

11. **Always Warm Up.** Don't take warming up lightly. It's necessary for:

• Reducing the risk of abnormal heartbeats
• Appropriate amounts of oxygen to be sent to the muscles (which occurs through gradual loosening of the muscles)
• Improved range-of-motion and balanced coordination
• Transition from inactivity to moderate or strenuous activity
• Preventing injuries

We'll provide you with some good warm-up techniques, but your entire warm up should last between ten and fifteen minutes, and should raise your pulse about five beats per minute.

12. Listen to your body. As you exercise, pay close attention to what's going on inside of your body. Remember, there's no need to feel extreme pain, so if you do, stop. If you feel mild pain, is it because your muscle isn't used to the exertion, or is it because you're pulling on it the wrong way? Maybe it's saying, "give me a rest!" With each step you take, each block you cycle around, each weight you lift, check in with yourself. Have you had enough? Can you do another lap? Before you know it, you'll be in tune with what your body needs. You may not always be able to accommodate what it communicates to you, but at least you will have established dialogue!

13. Start slowly. Begin your exercise program slowly and carefully. Starting slowly may mean doing a total of three repetitions with free weights or swimming for two minutes. If you do more than your body can handle, you may risk injury or you may not want to continue with the program.

14. Condition Yourself in Three-week Cycles. What were the most worthwhile accomplishments in your life? Chances are, they did not happen overnight. Nor will getting fit.

Once you start your routine, and if it feels right, stick with it for three weeks. Then evaluate whether or not you can increase your reps, cycle another mile, or walk a few more blocks. But stick with three-week increments because it takes about that long to reap the benefits of any given routine. If, however, at the end of the three-week period you aren't ready to do more, don't sweat! Give it another three weeks and then decide what's next.

EXERCISE TESTING

You may consider getting an exercise test before starting your regular exercise program. Even though you know you have OA, you may want to evaluate whether you have other, more subtle health conditions. Exercise testing, performed by doctors, physical therapists, and some certified physical fitness trainers, can determine:

• Cardiovascular health
• Muscular health
• Flexibility
• Body composition

15. Adjust Your Routine to You. It's wise to alternate the intensity of the workout so you can get to know your limits. Lighten up your routine on those days that you lack energy or go all out (without overdoing it) when you feel great. Other days you may think you're Superman or Wonder Woman in the flesh! Go for it! Observe what happens on both a physical and psychological level.

16. Keep Yourself Hydrated. You may not want to lug around a bottle of water while you exercise, but it may prevent you from becoming dizzy, disoriented, or falling and injuring yourself. Sports psychologist Tom Seabourne, M.D., suggests the following rules to keep yourself hydrated:

- Drink even when you are not thirsty. Older people especially need to force themselves to do this.
- Weigh yourself before and after exercise. Drink one pint (two cups) of liquid for each pound you have lost.
- Drink at least a cup of water one half hour before exercise.
- Don't drink or eat anything sugary within two hours before exercise.
- Drink three to six ounces of fluid every fifteen to twenty minutes during exercise that lasts longer than thirty minutes. Do this even if you're exercising in a cool room and don't feel yourself sweating or don't feel thirsty. If you wait until you are thirsty, you are already dehydrated.

AVOIDING CHARLEY HORSE

Most people know how suddenly and severely a muscle cramp, or Charley Horse, can occur. Typically, when you overexert a muscle it cramps up. To avoid muscle spasms during exercise, be sure to warm up before you undertake moderate or strenuous exercise; make sure you drink plenty of fluids so you don't become dehydrated; and ease up on working the muscle that's cramping. If you get muscle cramps at night (usually when contracting an overused muscle), try to relax the muscle, then massage it gently. If that doesn't help, try applying either heat or cold compresses.

- Drink cool fluids. They hydrate the body faster than warm or ice-cold beverages.
- After you exercise, drink sports drinks or fruit juice. They'll replenish your potassium and sodium levels that are sweat out during exercise and important to replace.

17. Keep Breathing. Most exercises will work more efficiently if you breathe properly. Breathing encourages your heart to pump adequate amounts of oxygen to your muscles during exercise. But how to breathe properly? It depends on what you're doing. If you're swimming, your breathing patterns will differ from when you're riding a bike or running. Be sure to consult with the professional you work with about the best way to breathe for your exercise of choice. When performing exercises, however, never hold your breath. Your body relies on the continuous cycle of incoming oxygen and outgoing carbon dioxide to function. Let your breathing naturally become faster as your heart rate increases. A general rule when working with weights is to exhale when you're pushing or lifting and inhale when you relax or release.

18. Monitor Your Heart Rate. According to the American Heart Association, you need to exercise for thirty to sixty minutes three to four times per week in order to reap the benefits of exercise, especially for the heart. If you exercise more than four times per week, it will increase those benefits. To do that, however, you need to increase your heart rate by 50 to 65 percent during exercise. Keep in mind, though, that intense aerobic exercises may be something you have to work toward. To estimate how to achieve 50 to 65 percent of your maximum heart rate, make the following calculations:

1. Subtract your age from 220. That amount equals your maximum heart rate.
2. Multiply that figure by 50 percent. That equals the lowest number of heartbeats you should reach while exercising.
3. Multiply your maximum heart rate by 65 percent. That equals

FINDING YOUR TARGET HEART RATE

Locate your pulse by placing one finger on either the radial artery (the underside of your wrist on the "thumbside"), or on the carotid artery (right side of your neck under your jaw, in alignment with the corner of your eye). Practice taking your heart rate before any activity or exercise so you're familiar with your pulse points. During aerobic exercise count the number of pulses you feel at your pulse point for six seconds and add a zero (which is the same as multiplying by ten) and you have your target heart rate. For a sixty-year-old exerciser, the number of pulses per six seconds should be between eight and ten.

the highest number of heartbeats you should reach while exercising.

For example, if you are sixty years old, the calculation will go as follows:

220 - 60 = 160
160 x 50% = 80 (beats per minute for the low end)
160 x 65% = 104 (beats per minute for the high end)

To achieve the benefits of exercise, your heart rate will have to reach at least 80 beats per minute, but should not exceed 104 beats per minute. Check your pulse after ten minutes of exercise to establish your heart rate. If it is below 80 beats per minute, you need to work a bit harder. If it exceeds 104 beats per minute, you need to ease up.

Another way to determine how you're exercising is by checking your breathing. If, while you bicycle or walk, you are comfortable and can talk with ease, you may want to push a little harder. Simply pick up the pace. If, on the other hand, you are gasping and unable to talk at all, you're pushing too hard. If you're breathing deeply but can speak in short sentences, you're probably right where you need to be. Check your heart rate every ten minutes or so during your workout, and then after you've finished. This will enable you to monitor your progress. As your cardiovascular health improves, you'll notice your resting heart rate will go down—a sure sign that exercise is helping your heart function more efficiently.

19. Cool Down. Few people know that if you had a choice of either warming up or cooling down, you should choose the latter. Cooling down enables your pulse to return to normal at a gradual pace. If you don't cool down, it can cause your heart to beat too quickly which can result in heart attack or irregular heart beats. Cooling down also prevents blood from pooling in your legs, a condition that can lead to dizziness, blackouts, and disorientation. A less alarming fact is that simple stretches after your workout will keep your muscles from cramping up, getting stiff, or becoming sore. You can do the same exercises that you warmed up with for your cool down, just at a slower pace and follow with some stretches.

20. **Record Your Workout and Give Yourself Credit.** Keep a journal of your workout and write down everything. Even if you had a bad workout, record what you did anyway and give yourself credit for what you *did* accomplish. Even if that means you did only one lap in the pool or three blocks on the bike. You did it even if it didn't match up to your expectation; in the long run it will contribute to your feeling better, losing weight, and improving your state of mind. Persistence, a positive attitude, and perseverance will bring you through on those bad workout days. If you had a great day, record that too, and acknowledge yourself for

WORKING OUT UP HIGH

Exercising at high altitudes (usually higher than 4500 feet above sea level) where the air is "thinner" means you'll have to breathe a little harder to get oxygen and your heart has to beat faster in order to get that oxygen to your muscles. Your body will tire sooner, as well. It probably means you'll tire sooner, too.

An increased heart rate and faster breathing is normal for people exercising in new high-altitude areas. But be aware that pushing too hard can spell disaster. High-altitude sickness is a serious condition that can be fatal—even for very fit people in their twenties. The symptoms include headache, nausea, and vomiting, loss of appetite, dizziness, insomnia, and an overall feeling of illness. Don't mistake these symptoms for the flu. If you experience them while at high altitude, call a doctor immediately.

It takes a good eight days for the body to adapt to thin air, so if you're at a high altitude while vacationing, for example, don't expect to accomplish what you do at home. Take it slow and easy, knowing that you'll be home soon and can resume your regular exercise routine.

attaining or exceeding your goals. Reward yourself by buying some flowers, going to a movie, or calling a loved one long distance and sharing the good news.

THE WRONG WAY TO A GOOD
EXERCISE PROGRAM

When it comes to starting an exercise program it is wise to use common sense. For instance, if you have painful OA in your wrist and it hurts terribly when you apply sudden pressure to it, don't take up a racquet sport. Instead try some easy isometric stretches, coupled with brisk aerobic walks, and a yoga class. Perhaps your knee is what troubles you—then, a game of football, basketball, or hockey is probably not a good idea. Rather, engage in some dynamic stretches, water aerobics, and three or four bike rides per week. If you've recently incurred an injury, wait until it has *completely* healed before you begin your routine.

This may sound rudimentary but sometimes overenthusiasm or impatience causes us to do things that may worsen our condition. In the following, we debunk some common exercise myths.

Myth #1—Go for the pain! No pain, no gain! Wrong! You may feel some pressure or light burning that you're not accustomed to when starting an exercise program, but that doesn't mean you should be in pain. If you feel pain during exercise—stop! Do not

MUSIC MAKES THE DIFFERENCE

A preliminary study conducted on twenty-five OA women ranging in age from sixty-five to ninety-nine years of age showed that listening to fast-paced jazz music while doing repetitive exercises increased the number of repetitions performed.

Need a little motivation to complete your reps? Pull out the Count Basie, Frank Sinatra, Elvis, the Rolling Stones—anything that gets you motivated—and watch yourself pump. Or, if you need to pick up the pace while on your walks, shop around for a Walkman. Put in your favorite music, plug in the tiny headphones, and boogie your way to the one-mile marker.

"work through the pain"—especially if your pain is coming from your arthritic joint.

Muscle soreness, which may occur, is caused by lactic acid build up in the muscle. This is a natural occurrence when exercising—you'll only "feel" it when you overuse a muscle. As you exercise you will notice the difference between muscle fatigue from challenging or building a muscle and arthritic pain. Listen to your body and pay attention to the type of pain you're feeling, and respond to it accordingly.

Myth #2—Exercising on Hard Surfaces is Fine. Not if you're attempting to heal an arthritic joint! In fact, consistently running or playing on hard surfaces may cause new problems—especially if you're wearing worn shoes. Look for softer surfaces like grass or a local track on which to walk or run, and a carpeted, wood, or matted floor for a dance or aerobics class.

Myth #3—Eat, Breathe, and Sleep, Exercise! Obsessing can be dangerous. Remember, fitness is a three-dimensional goal. An exercise program should not *take over* your life. Take a step back and make sure you're not going overboard.

Myth #4—Stick with the Program, Even if You're Sick. Take care of yourself when you're sick. You can get back on track when you're feeling well again. It may mean losing a little strength or flexibility, but you won't enjoy exercise when you're sick, and what your body needs is rest.

Myth #5—Eat Whatever You Want Because You'll Burn it Off. Even if you don't need to lose weight, your physical well-being is dependent on intelligent portions of healthy food. In the Arthritis Cure Fitness Plan, eating and exercise work hand-in-hand.

EXERCISE AND WEIGHT LOSS:
THE PERFECT MARRIAGE

The overwhelming number of people who have OA are overweight. That's often the reason their joints have worn down; they simply weren't made to carry the extra pounds. Even though weight loss may be something you've battled with for a long time, in order to achieve a pain-free, healthy life, you must face the weight and reasons why you have it—and lose it once and for all. If you have medical conditions that contribute to your weight problem, speak frankly with your doctor and ask for direction on how to lose it. Weight loss is an enormous part of bringing your body, mind, and spirit into balance.

To bring yourself back to a reasonable weight that will help relieve your joints of the pressure they've been under, exercise—especially aerobics and strength training as through the Arthritis Cure Fitness Plan—is the most effective way. And, unlike dieting alone, exercise enables you to shed 100 percent fat. Dieting may cause weight loss, too, but about one third of what you lose may be muscle. If you want to lose weight *you need to commit to both a good eating plan and regular exercise.*

Time. That's what losing weight takes. And perseverance. The longer you've carried excess weight, the longer it will take to lose it because your metabolism is slower and takes longer to burn calories—your body is accustomed to storing calories rather than burning them. It may take as much time to lose weight as it did to gain it.

But don't distress. The most important thing to keep in mind is that exercise *will* change your metabolism and allow you to burn fat and lose weight.

Simply, to lose weight, your body must burn more calories than it takes in (one pound=3500 calories). The more activities you do in a day, the more calories you burn.

As you design your fitness program, keep in mind that if you can't squeeze in an hour's worth of exercise at one time, you can break it into two thirty-minute routines, or four fifteen-minute programs. There's always a way to make it work. But no matter how old you are, how overweight you are, or how long you've been overweight, aerobics and strength training will help you burn calories quicker than anything else.

As time goes on and you lose weight, your metabolism will become more efficient, making it easier and easier to lose weight.

As part of the Arthritis Cure Fitness Plan, we urge you to stay apprised of the latest breaking news, whether it's about how to exercise, what to eat, or tips on how to keep an open mind. To that end, consider subscribing to a few magazines like *Cooking Light, Shape, Self,* or *Modern Maturity.* They'll keep you posted, through simple, easy-to-read articles, about what the myriad studies on health are revealing, and maybe provide you with some good, low-fat recipes, and inspiration along the way!

CHAPTER FIVE

The Arthritis Cure Fitness Plan—Let's Go!

"I don't deserve this award, but I have arthritis and I don't deserve that either."

—JACK BENNY

THE ARTHRITIS CURE FITNESS PLAN (ACFP) incorporates warm-up/cool down exercises, stretching, muscle strengthening, and aerobic exercises. These exercises can be done at home or at a gym. Either way, we suggest consulting a fitness expert to ensure that you're doing them correctly. The ACFP is based on a four-week program and builds gradually. By the fourth week you will have built an exercise program catered to your own specific needs. Continue exercising from that level and increase the level as your body becomes more conditioned. We suggest adding some fun, recreational activities to your week; for instance, gardening, playing with your dog, or taking your grandchildren to the park. Also, yoga (see Chapter 6) is an excellent source of relaxation and will increase your flexibility.

Monitor your progress. Many people like to give themselves the weekend off, while others use Saturday and Sunday to make up for the times they missed during the week. Do what works for you.

WEEK I: WARM-UP/COOL DOWN
Do these simple warm-up/cool down exercises twice a day, five days a week. These exercises are for the total body, so be sure to do them slowly and with control. If you experience pain, take it easy and

only push it as far as you can without straining yourself. You can do most of the following warm-up/cool down exercises either standing tall or sitting upright in a chair.

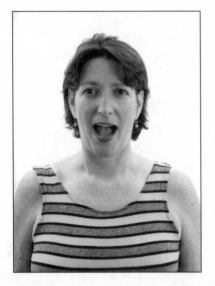

FACE

Move every muscle in your face with exaggerated movements. Say the five vowels this way to invigorate the facial muscles. Don't forget to move your eyebrows, tongue, ears, and nose. After your face feels "awake" move on to your neck.

NECK

Look left and right slowly, several times. Then drop your head to your left shoulder (ear to shoulder), your chest (chin to chest), and your right shoulder (ear to shoulder). *Do not drop your head back.* Repeat these movements eight to ten times or until your neck muscles feel loose.

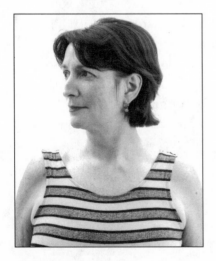

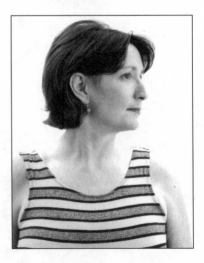

FINGERS, HANDS, WRISTS

Bend your fingers, then splay them out wide. Repeat. Hold your right hand out flat, palm up. Take your left hand and gently press down on your right fingers. You'll feel a good stretch in your wrist. Now press on the back of your hand so your fingers reach toward your inner wrist. Repeat on the other hand. Flex your wrists forward and back; then circle them. Reverse the circles.

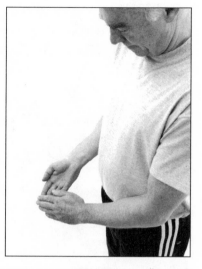

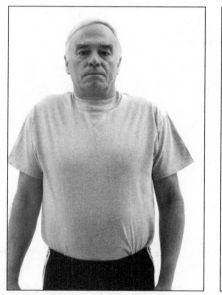
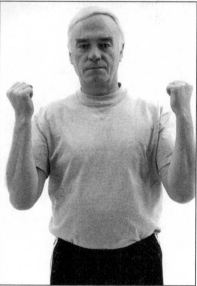

ARMS AND SHOULDERS

Shrug your shoulders (lift and release). Push them back, then pull them forward. Then move them in a circular motion (up, back, down, and forward in smooth circles). Do eight to ten circles back; reverse and do them forward.

Starting with your arms at your sides, bend your elbows bringing

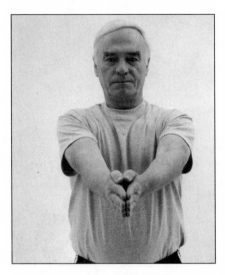

your fists to your shoulders. Repeat eight to ten times. Touch your palms together in front of you, then open your arms with palms down as wide as they'll go (like the wings of an airplane). With your arms open as wide as they'll go, turn palms up and raise your hands above your head, clasping hands at the top and making your arms into a point. Release your hands and make big circles with your arms (up, back, down, and forward in smooth circles). Circle eight to ten

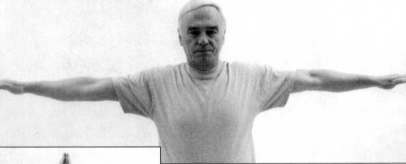

times backward; then reverse and circle eight to ten times forward.

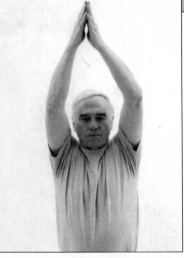

EXERCISE AND THE NATURAL "HIGH"

After about thirty-five minutes of aerobic exercise—walking, running, cycling, swimming, dancing, etc.—tiny peptide molecules, called endorphins, in your brain become activated. Their job? They bind themselves to pain receptors in your brain, reducing the feeling of pain. These molecules not only numb physical pain, but also

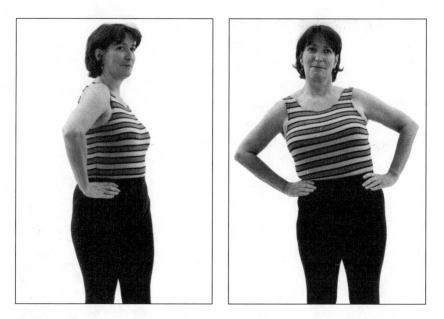

TORSO

(It is more effective to stand while doing these warm-up exercises.)

With your hands on your hips, twist from the waist to the left and hold for five seconds; then twist to the right and hold. Repeat one time. Keeping your hips stationery, bring your rib cage forward, right, back, and left making smooth circles with your rib cage. Circle four times to the right; then reverse and circle four times to the left. Then bend to the right from the waist, bend forward, and bend left. Reverse. Repeat four times. *Do not bend back.*

emotional pain like anxiety or depression. That's evidence that moderate or vigorous exercise really *can* boost your self-esteem. Serious runners and joggers have coined the phrase "runner's high" from the morphine-like effect of the endorphins. Even if you take a brisk thirty-five minute walk three to five days a week, you'll experience the equivalent of taking eight mg. of morphines. (Even a good session of yoga can activate the reaction.) Studies also show that once the endorphins come into play, emotions become stabilized for the rest of the day. So, if you wake up on the wrong side of the bed, go out for thirty-five minutes of aerobic exercise; chances are you'll be smiling until you turn in at the end of the day.

Buttocks and Hips

In a standing position, squeeze the buttocks and release. Squeeze and release eight to ten times. Keeping your upper body, waist, and legs stationery, make circles with your hips bringing them, forward, right, back, and left. Do four circles to the right. Reverse and do four circles to the left.

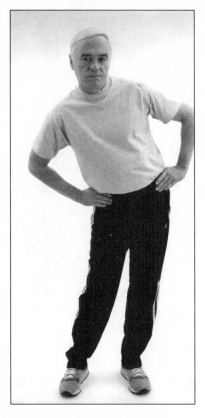

Legs

Start in a seated position, which protects your back. With one leg firmly planted, bring your other knee to your chest by placing your hands behind the knee and pulling it towards your body. Repeat on the other side, hold for 10 seconds to feel the stretch. Sitting with both

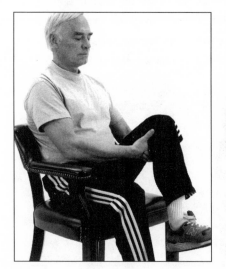

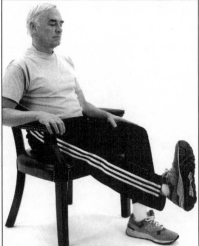

feet on the floor, raise one foot to knee level, straightening your leg and flexing toes to the ceiling. Don't strain yourself; just lift to where you feel it stretch. You should feel the stretch in the back of your thigh, knee, and calf. Slowly and with control, drop your leg. Repeat with the other leg. Do eight to ten repetitions for each leg. While sitting, do ankle circles. Also gently point and flex your toes.

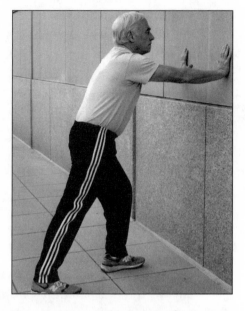

Standing about two feet from a wall, lean in and place both hands on the wall in front of you. Straighten one leg pressing your heel to the floor, and keep the other bent. Hold for eight seconds and repeat. You will feel the stretch along the back of your leg and calf. Hold for about twenty seconds, then switch legs.

IF YOU HAVE BEEN SEDENTARY for a long time, start slowly and steadily. Don't push it. Do whatever you can to support yourself emotionally and physically. For Week I do the complete warm-up/cool down exercises twice a day (we suggest in the morning upon waking, and at night before bed), for five days. (Once we add muscle strengthening and cardio to your workout, in Weeks III and IV, you should do these exercises immediately before your workout as a warm-up and immediately after as a cool down).

	MON.	TUES.	WED.	THURS.	FRI.	SAT.	SUN.
WEEK I	AM: warm-up/cool down PM: warm-up/cool down	AM: warm-up/cool down PM: warm-up/cool down	AM: warm-up/cool down PM: warm-up/cool down	AM: warm-up/cool down PM: warm-up/cool down	AM: warm-up/cool down PM: warm-up/cool down	Recreation	Rest

WEEK II: Stretching

For Week II of the Arthritis Cure Fitness Plan add stretching for flexibility to your workout once a day for five days. For your first couple of days you may want to pick one stretch from either upper body or lower body stretches. You'll notice that, combined with your warm-up/cool down exercises, after about your second week you'll feel much more confident and may be ready to do all the stretches. If you feel ready to do all the stretches your second week, go right ahead. As you exercise regularly, you will find that stretching will not only increase your flexibility, but will also reduce the discomfort of muscle exertion.

UPPER BODY STRETCHES
Chest

Show Off: From a standing position, place your hands behind your back and clasp them together. If you can't grasp your hands together

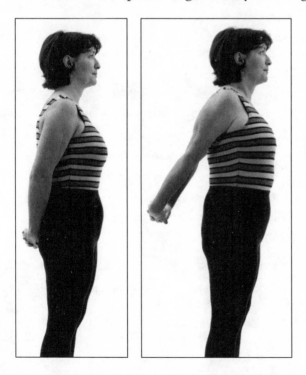

behind you, grab onto a towel or elastic band with both hands. Then, as though you want to flaunt your favorite necklace or necktie, pull back your shoulders while lifting your hands a few inches higher. Your chest will automatically expand. Hold for ten to thirty seconds.

NECK

Oh-So-Coy Neck Stretch: Either sit or stand to do this one. Slowly drop your right ear to your right shoulder (but don't lift your shoulder) and simply hold it for ten to thirty seconds. Then lower your chin straight down to your chest and hold it there for ten to thirty seconds. Finally, lift your chin so your left ear reaches for your left shoulder. Hold that for ten to thirty seconds. You can use your opposite hand to gently push your neck closer to your shoulder. *Be absolutely certain not to drop your head back or to do a complete circle with your neck. Alternate only from one side, forward, and then to the next side—never drop the weight of your head to the back.*

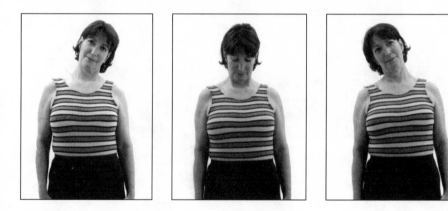

BACK AND TORSO

Angel Trunk Twist: Lay flat on your back. Press your lower back to the floor so that your back is not arched. Lift your knees and slowly lower them to your left side so that your right knee and ankle rests on your left knee and ankle. Spread your arms out to your side like angel wings so they're level with your shoulders. Turn your head to the opposite direction of your knees. Make sure your shoulders are flat on the floor, or as close to flat as possible. Relax into the stretch. Stay in that position for thirty seconds, more if you feel yourself stretching more. Then repeat the stretch gently easing your legs to the right side, turning your head to the left. You'll feel this gentle, soothing twist in your back and legs.

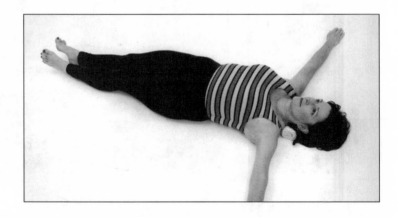

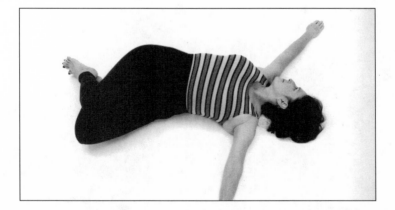

Hunting Dog Pose: Get on your hands and knees, making sure your hands are directly below your shoulders, and your knees directly below your hips. Keep your back and neck straight (don't arch or round it) so your head is held and eyes looking down at the floor. Keep your stomach muscles taut so they support your back. Slowly and gently raise

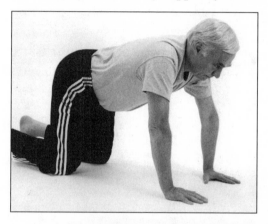

your right foot straight behind you with your toes flexed slightly, so your leg is parallel to the floor. Then, take your opposite hand, or left hand, and put it straight out before you. Hold for ten to thirty seconds. Repeat using opposite leg and hand.

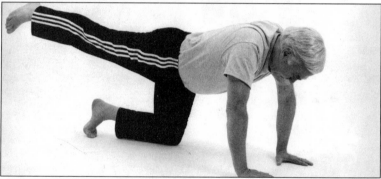

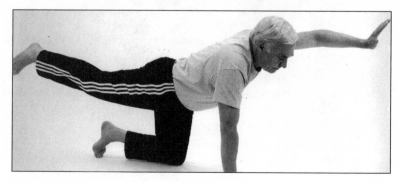

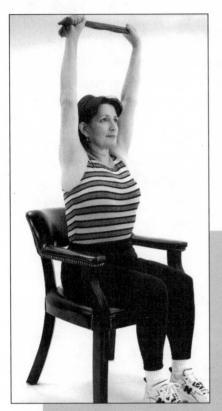

SHOULDERS

Shoulder Cobra: Either sitting or standing, reach for the sky and lift the upper trunk of your body as high as it can go. After ten seconds, clasp your hands together (use a towel or elastic band if necessary), palms upward, and reach even higher while bringing your elbows to your ears. Hold ten to twenty more seconds.

GET CRACKING WITH A CHIROPRACTOR

Chiropractic care has been around since 1895, and is conducted by licensed practitioners who base their work on spinal and joint manipulation. They utilize X rays if an area is seriously injured, but they have several other means of determining what may be causing the discomfort.

Chiropractors usually consider the entire body as well as external forces while making their diagnosis and deciding on treatment. That means they may look carefully at posture, diet, stress, and general physical well-being.

The "adjustments" are made on a chiropractic table with the doctor's hands or instruments made specifically for their purposes. The adjustments generally don't hurt, although they can cause some loud cracking noises from nitrogen that erupts from the joints.

As with any newly developed ache or pain, be sure you are addressing the real issue and seeking appropriate care. If you break your ankle, go to a medical doctor, not a chiropractor. If, however, you find a new ache somewhere in your body that seems like it's a result of your new routine, try chiropractic care. They have also been known to provide relief to those who suffer with OA. As always, don't stick with a practitioner whom you don't like or that doesn't provide results within a given amount of time.

UPPER ARM AND BACK

Triceps Stretch: Stand about three feet from the corner of a wall. Bend your right arm and place your right elbow on the wall. Step forward, past the wall, with your left foot as if you were doing a partial lunge. As your chest leans towards the wall, you will feel a stretch in your triceps, along the bottom of your arm. Repeat with other arm.

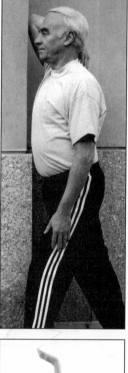

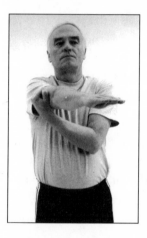

Lazy Arm: Cross your right arm over your chest and grab the upper part of it with your left hand so it completely supports your right arm. Hold the "lazy arm" and gently pull on it to stretch the upper shoulder. Hold for ten to thirty seconds and repeat on opposite side.

TORSO

Atlas Shrug: Stand up, legs slightly apart, weight distributed evenly over hips. Place your left hand firmly on the outside of your left thigh, and raise your right hand, palm to the sky (as if you're holding a globe), high above your head. Gently lean the weight of your torso over your left hip, leading with your right hand. Keep your hip stable and steady, and only go as far as you can so you feel a stretch on the right side of your body. Then hold steady (don't shrug) for ten to thirty seconds. Repeat on the opposite side.

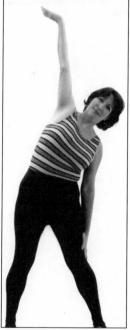

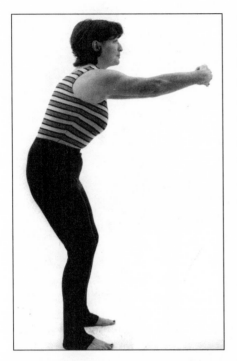

UPPER BACK

Tug 'O War: Standing with feet slightly apart, lace your fingers and extend arms straight in front of your chest. Push outwardly, as if a rope was pulling you, so your upper back and shoulders round forward. Continue your back stretch by rotating pelvis slightly forward so your entire back is slightly rounded. Hold ten to thirty seconds.

LOWER BODY STRETCHES
HAMSTRING (Back of Thigh)

One Leg Up: Stand up and hold onto a supportive surface like a banister, table, or countertop; keep one foot on the floor and place the other on an elevated surface like a stair or stool. Slowly lean forward, bringing your chest to your knee. Lean just until you feel the stretch in the back of your thigh. Once you feel the stretch, hold for five seconds and repeat on other side.

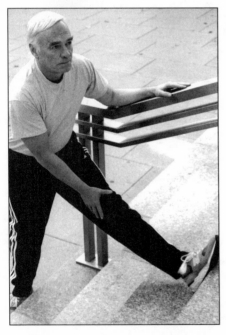

Leaning Tower: Seated in a sturdy chair, sit on the edge of it with your hands on your hips. Then straighten your right leg in front of you while keeping your left leg bent. Lean forward from the hips, bringing the chest towards the knee, and you'll feel a good stretch behind your right leg. Hold for ten to thirty seconds, and repeat on the opposite side. Feel the stretch in the back of your thigh, knee, and calf.

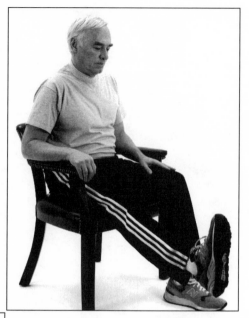

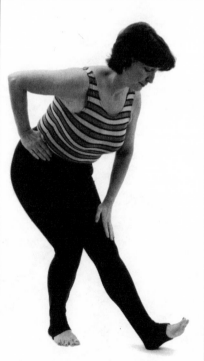

Royal Curtsy: Stand up straight, feet directly beneath hips. Bend both knees, and then straighten left leg by putting it forward, flexing your foot so the heel rests on the floor. Keep your right knee bent. Then slowly lean forward from the hip. Bend until you feel a good stretch on the back of the thigh of your left leg. Hold for ten to thirty seconds. Repeat other side.

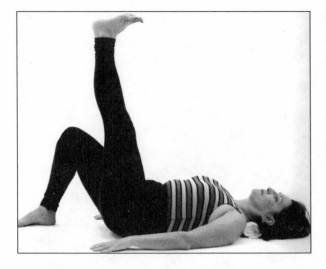

QUADRICEPS
(Front of Thigh)

Robot Leg: You can do this sitting on a chair or lying on the floor. Simply extend your left leg straight in front of you (if you're sitting) or straight above you (if you're lying down) and hold it there for a count of ten. Repeat the exercise as many times as you comfortably can; try to work up to at least ten times. Do the same with your right leg. This is especially good if the arthritis is in your knees.

Flamingo: Standing straight and tall, use your left hand to grasp the back of a chair, or lean against a wall or some other stationary object. Then bend the right leg, lifting your foot behind you. Grasp your right ankle with your right hand, making certain that your back is straight, not arched, and pull your right heel into your buttocks. You'll feel a good stretch on your upper right thigh. Keep your right knee close to your other leg so it doesn't travel out to the side. Hold for ten to thirty seconds and repeat on the opposite side. This will stretch the front of your thigh and hip.

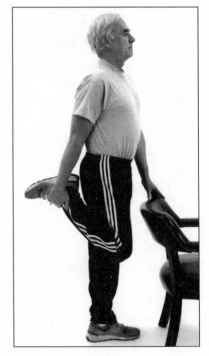

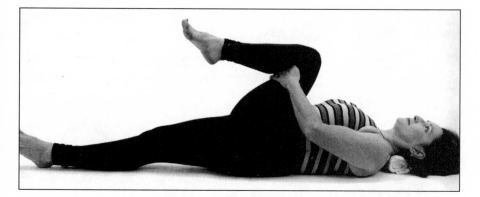

BUTTOCKS

Knee-Chest Kiss: Lie flat on floor with knee bent, or sit on a chair. Lift right leg up, and grasp under the knee with your hands. Gently and slowly raise the knee to your chest as far as you can. If possible, bring the knee all the way to your chest, as if they're going to kiss. Hold for ten to thirty seconds. Repeat with left leg. This will loosen your back and buttocks.

Sitting Knee Hold: Sitting up straight in a chair, place your left ankle on your right knee. This is the position many people use to cross their legs. Now, simply push down on your left knee and you'll feel the stretch in your upper legs and buttocks. Hold for twenty seconds and switch sides.

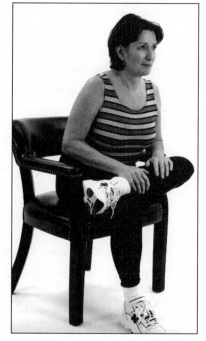

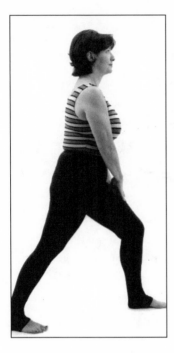

CALF

On Your Mark, Get Set! Step forward with your left foot as if you're queuing for a big race. Move your weight over your left leg, but bend your left-knee slightly so as not to cause undo strain. Keep your right heel on the floor and feel the stretch in that calf as you lean forward. Hold ten to thirty seconds. Repeat on the opposite side.

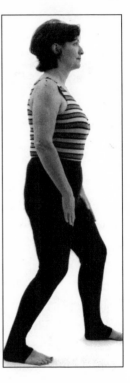

Flat Foot Calf Stretch: Stand straight with weight over hips. Step forward with left foot, but keep your right heel on the floor. Slowly bend both knees and move pelvis forward to stretch lower part of right calf. Hold ten to thirty seconds. Switch sides.

	MON.	TUES.	WED.	THURS.	FRI.	SAT.	SUN.
WEEK I	AM: warm-up/cool down PM: warm-up/cool down	AM: warm-up/cool down PM: warm-up/cool down	AM: warm-up/cool down PM: warm-up/cool down	AM: warm-up/cool down PM: warm-up/cool down	AM: warm-up/cool down PM: warm-up/cool down	Recreation	Rest
WEEK II	AM: warm-up/cool down; stretching PM: warm-up/cool down	AM: warm-up/cool down; stretching PM: warm-up/cool down	AM: warm-up/cool down; stretching PM: warm-up/cool down	AM: warm-up/cool down; stretching PM: warm-up/cool down	AM: warm-up/cool down; stretching PM: warm-up/cool down	Yoga	Rest

WEEK III: MUSCLE STRENGTHENING

Most of the following exercises make use of an elastic band or rubber tube that provides resistance, but it is possible to do them without weights, letting gravity be your resistance. You can buy elastic bands at pharmacies or sporting good stores, or save money and use a bike tire inner tube that you can customize, cut, and tie together (make sure it has no cracks). Free weights or dumbbells are available at sporting good stores, come in all different sizes and weights, and don't cost much. Even so, you can make your own by placing rice or pennies into an old sock. Place it on your bathroom scale to make sure you have the appropriate weight.

It's always best to begin any exercise without weights until you achieve the number of repetitions you want to do. Then add one or two pounds, increasing in practical increments, or add repetitions. You know you're using the proper weight if after about eight to ten repetitions of the exercise you feel a slight burning sensation in the muscle you are working—this is how you challenge and strengthen your muscles. Be mindful of your level of fitness and condition of

A BEDROOM SCENE

Most of the warm-up/cool down exercises of the Arthritis Cure Fitness Plan can be done from the comfort of your bed. It's cozy, you're warm from being there all night, and you're feeling relaxed. Even though you may be stiff, you can still limber yourself up right then and there: Begin by wiggling your toes, flexing and gently pointing your feet, and doing "circles" with your ankles. Traveling up your body, flex and relax your calf muscles and quadriceps. After that, bend your knees, lift one leg, stretch it, and draw "leg circles" in the air; then do the other leg. (Never lift both legs at once.) Keep your knees bent while you then try some gentle twisting at your waist. Still with knees bent, grasp the back of your thighs or your knees and do a single sit up, lifting just your upper body. Release. Move your hands, arms, and fingers any way you can, being mindful of painful limitations. Finally, move your head from side to side on the pillow to get your neck muscles ready for the day. By now, you're ready to rise—and you may not even need a cup of coffee.

OA, and don't take on more weight then you can handle. Slowly build up to a weight you want to lift. A good rule is: Don't use weights that exceed 10 percent of your total body weight for each limb.[1]

We suggest doing the muscle strengthening exercises at least three times a week for best results. Do the warm-up/cool down exercises before and after muscle strengthening. In Week IV we will alternate muscle strengthening with cardio for the complete Arthritis Cure Fitness Plan.

UPPER BODY EXERCISES

Directing Traffic: Raise arms straight above your head, and then slowly drop them to the side. Next, bend your elbows so your fists are at your shoulders. Then straighten them out again. Do eight to ten repetitions, and increase weight or repetitions over time. Do this exercise with or without weights (tip: in place of weights use two full cans of food in each hand). Strengthens shoulders and biceps.

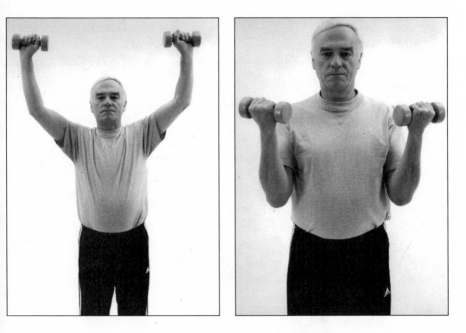

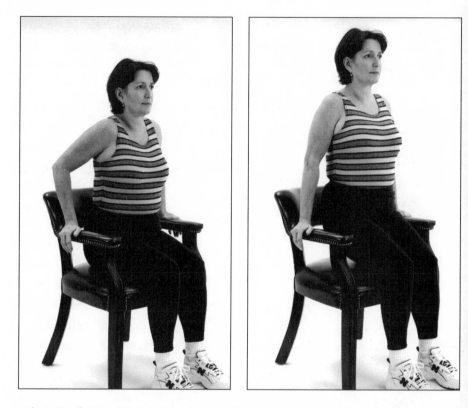

Chair Push Ups: Sit in a sturdy armchair, then push yourself up with your arms only (no leg power). Repeat eight to ten times. Strengthens shoulders and triceps. *This is beneficial for those wanting to increase their upper body strength, but should not be done by those with problem hands or wrists.*

KEEPING YOUR RESISTANCE BAND IN SHAPE

Look at the band carefully for weakened areas that might tear during exercise. The band is sturdy but not impenetrable. Keep sharp objects away from it, and don't use it while wearing jewelry. Don't leave the band in direct sunlight. Heat can dry it out and weaken it. Protect it by rubbing talcum powder on it. Securely tie the band with a knot or bow before you begin your program. Then, untie it when you're finished. Don't stretch the band more than ten to fifteen feet. It could snap during use and cause extreme pain or injury.[2]

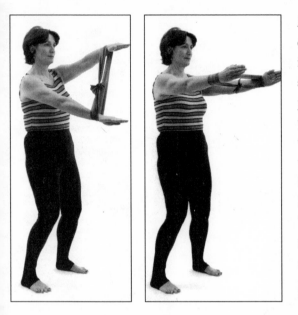

Butterfly Net: Place the elastic band around your forearms. Extend your arms out straight with palms down. Don't bend your elbows. Push down with one arm and pull up with the other. Hold for five seconds then relax. Repeat on opposite side. With the elastic band still around your forearms, straighten arms with palms facing each other. Then, move arms out to the side until belt is tight. Hold for five seconds. Repeat eight to ten times. Strengthens front shoulder and chest muscles.

LOWER BODY EXERCISES

Foot Flex: Laying flat on your back, bend your right knee. Flex your left foot, and with a straight leg, raise it slightly, no more than six inches. Hold for ten seconds. Repeat on opposite side. Start slowly but try increasing to eight to twelve repetitions for each leg. Strengthens quadriceps (front of thigh).

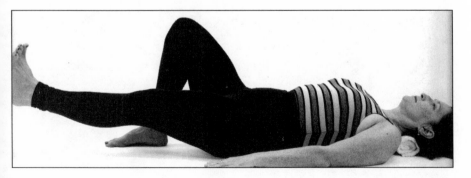

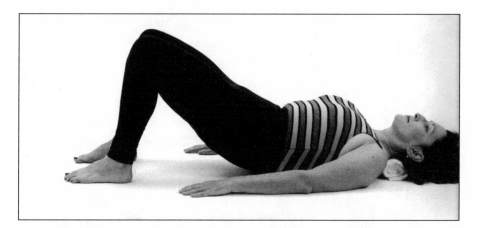

Half Pyramid: While lying on your back, bend both knees. Then, pushing from your feet, raise your buttocks three or four inches. Hold it for ten seconds. Slowly release, and lay flat for five seconds. Repeat this eight to twelve times. Strengthens quadriceps (front of thigh).

Leg Pulley: Sitting in a chair or lying on the floor, place the elastic band around your ankles, with knees straight. Spread your legs slowly as you push against the belt. Hold for ten seconds. Repeat eight to twelve times. Strengthens outer thigh or hips.

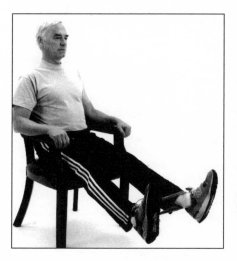
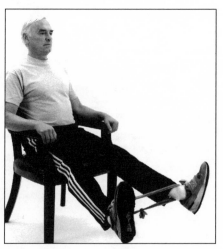

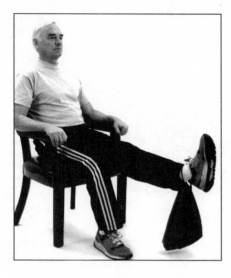

Bag Drag: Sit in a chair and place the handles of a plastic grocery bag that contains one or two full cans around your right ankle. Then lift your left leg straight in front of you, pulling the bag up with you. Hold and count to five. Slowly put your foot down, and repeat for as many times as you can until you can do eight to ten times. Repeat on opposite side. This is an excellent exercise for strengthening quadriceps to relieve stress to your knee joint.

	MON.	TUES.	WED.	THURS.	FRI.	SAT.	SUN.
WEEK I	AM: warm-up/cool down PM: warm-up/cool down	AM: warm-up/cool down PM: warm-up/cool down	AM: warm-up/cool down PM: warm-up/cool down	AM: warm-up/cool down PM: warm-up/cool down	AM: warm-up/cool down PM: warm-up/cool down	Recreation	Rest
WEEK II	AM: warm-up/cool down; stretching PM: warm-up/cool down	AM: warm-up/cool down; stretching PM: warm-up/cool down	AM: warm-up/cool down; stretching PM: warm-up/cool down	AM: warm-up/cool down; stretching PM: warm-up/cool down	AM: warm-up/cool down; stretching PM: warm-up/cool down	Yoga	Rest
WEEK III	WHOLE WORKOUT ANYTIME: warm-up/cool down; stretching; muscle strengthening; warm-up/cool down	AM: warm-up/cool down; stretching PM: warm-up/cool down	WHOLE WORKOUT ANYTIME: warm-up/cool down; stretching; muscle strengthening; warm-up/cool down	AM: warm-up/cool down; stretching PM: warm-up/cool down	WHOLE WORKOUT ANYTIME: warm-up/cool down; stretching; muscle strengthening; warm-up/cool down	Recreation	Rest

WEEK IV: CARDIOVASCULAR WORKOUTS

It's time to get your blood circulating and your heart pumping. You can do these workouts at a gym on treadmills, stationary bikes, or other equipment, or purchase equipment for your home use. What's great about cardiovascular workouts is you can take to the outdoors. Whichever you choose, be sure to get expert advice from a qualified trainer or fitness expert before you get started—if you are using equipment ask them how best to use it.

Alternate your cardio workouts with muscle strengthening and do them two to three times per week. Do the warm-up/cool down exercises before and after each cardio workout, and don't forget to monitor your progress.

Experiment with your cardiovascular workouts by trying the following exercises. Remember, working out doesn't need to be aggressive or overly strenuous. Just by getting your heart rate up for a defined period of time (fifteen to thirty minutes), you'll be strengthening your cardiovascular system and giving yourself the gift of better health.

All of the cardiovascular exercises described in this chapter can be safely done with arthritis. It is wise, however, to speak with your doctor or health care professional before beginning any workout program. Additionally, if your arthritis is focused in

GET HELP TO HIPS

Hip joints are the strongest in our body. Through simple, daily activities alone, they sustain up to six times their weight. Just think what they bear when we're running, dancing, or aerobicizing. As strong as they are, however, falls can occur. Whether you're in the kitchen, poolside, on the golf course, or walking in the woods, keep these things in mind:

If you fall or twist and feel pain in your hip area, call for help immediately. Since this is such a crucial joint, it must be attended to wisely and carefully. Serious pain and immobility signals either a dislocation or fracture and you will need urgent medical care.

If, after an evaluation from a doctor, you are only bruised, ice the area regularly for several days. It will reduce pain and swelling. If you've pulled a tendon, follow your doctor's instructions, and be mindful that it can take up to three months to recover completely. Don't push it. You'll heal eventually, but proper healing is key so you can resume your everyday life without harming yourself further.

one or more areas, you should consult with a fitness expert who understands your health needs and can help you tailor these exercises to your body.

WALKING

Walking may not be your first choice for an aerobic exercise, but it just may be the best. It's relatively easy, you don't need any equipment other than good shoes, you can do it alone or with others, and it provides as many cardiovascular benefits as running or jogging, minus the stress to your lower body.

Walking is gaining more and more attention because the more we learn about it, the more we realize that it's nature's near-perfect gift for good health. Plus it's simple to do. If you're an outdoor enthusiast, you can wind your way through the woods, do laps around a lake, hike up some hills, glide through a garden, or even fly around a football field. Nature provides every arena for those who love the great outdoors.

If it's cold and wintry outside and you don't feel like bundling up, you can drive to the mall, lace up your shoes, and cruise around without getting frostbite. If there isn't a mall nearby, check out one of the

WHEN TO SEEK PHYSICAL THERAPY

If you haven't already worked with an occupational or physical therapist to help you learn to manage your daily activities, you might consider doing so. Especially if you find it painful to do simple things like fastening buttons, putting on shoes, waiting in line, or reaching for something in a cupboard.

Both types of therapists can educate you on how to properly use helpful devices such as canes or long-handled shoehorns. They can also advise you about products developed solely for people with OA that enable you to utilize larger joints and muscles so you can relieve pain on smaller ones, for example, in your hands.

The Arthritis Foundation also sponsors Arthritis Self-Management Courses throughout the country. They will not only provide you with valuable information, but you might meet the perfect exercise buddy, or a new group of friends who understand your questions and concerns.

superstores in your area. Some grocery stores are big enough to add mileage to your soles, while discount stores or other mega-stores provide plenty of space for brisk walking that increases your heart rate and lubricates your joints.

Walking has also been targeted as one of the activities women can do to keep osteoporosis at bay. That's because it actually builds bone mass. That, coupled with calcium, can do wonders for postmenopausal women, as well as younger women who want to help increase their chances of a healthier, more upright old age.

If you've been sedentary for years and are just beginning to work out, walking may be the easiest exercise to integrate into your life. If you're up against terrible pain, take it as slowly as you need to. Remember that when walking, your stride should be heel-to-toe, you should not land on the ball of your foot first. Also, let your arms swing naturally, i.e. your opposite arm swings when you step forward.

Start by walking as far as you can—even if that only means to the end of the block and back again, two to three times a week. After a while, flexibility will return to your joints, and you might find that you could walk two blocks, then three. But take your time. There's no rush, and you don't want to do too much too soon.

HEALING THE HEEL

If you find yourself loving your aerobics class, but start to develop pain in your heel, be aware of this:

Sometimes heel pain indicates the development of a heel or bone spur, also known as plantar fasciitis. That happens when the fibrous tissue that runs along the arch of your foot becomes inflamed and isn't properly cared for. If you feel pain in your foot upon getting out of bed in the morning, and if it slowly fades throughout the day, but returns upon participating in the class, consider stopping the class for a week or so to see what happens.

You're more apt to get a bone spur if you have flat feet or pronation, knock-knees, or high arches. Also, neglecting to warm up before your aerobics class can cause tightening in your calf muscles which can also contribute to the condition.

As you take time off from the class, apply ice to the sore spot and massage it regularly. Consider purchasing orthotics for your exercise shoes, and avoid walking around without shoes. If, after about a week, you see no improvement, call your doctor for advice. You may need to alternate between aerobics and non-weight bearing exercises like swimming or cycling.

If you've been exercising moderately already, then try walking briskly for twenty minutes, two to three times a week. Increase your mileage and frequency as your body allows. Strive for at least thirty minutes a session, more if possible. That way you can reap the most benefits for your heart and joints, as well as get a boost from those mind-altering endorphins.

If you need inspiration, don't forget your best friend. Your dog could provide you with both more reason to go, and a smile to get into a new walking routine.

WRITE YOUR WAY TO FITNESS

It is important as part of the Arthritis Cure Fitness Team and to prepare for the mental and physical challenge of the Arthritis Cure Fitness Plan to keep a journal. It's a necessary tool for keeping track of your attitude, progress, fears and doubts, feelings about certain activities, and more. You can complain or rejoice—but as you write, you'll get to know yourself better and become aware of what's going on within you while recording the progress you make outwardly.

Following are the items to record as part of the Arthritis Cure Fitness Plan:

• How much do you weigh?

• What is your optimum weight?

• What are your measurements (upper arm, chest, waist, hips, thighs)?

• Where do you feel the most pain in your body? Where do you feel other aches and pains?

• When is the pain at its worst? Are there physical or emotional stresses that make it worse? If so, what are they?

• What kinds of physical activities do you do on a daily basis? What kind of exercise, if any, do you do, and for how long?

• Are you generally a happy person, depressed person, or somewhere in between? What makes you feel that way?

• What could you do today to feel better?

If, after you've answered these questions, you want to write more, go ahead and do it. Remember, the purpose of the journal is to record physical changes and experiences, but also, to provide a place in which you can vent, express, rant, cheer, explore—anything you want to do to keep the emotional, mental, and spiritual channels clear.

Walking is especially beneficial to those with OA in the hips, knees, and ankles, but it also helps if the joints in your back or neck are affected. Before walking, be sure to stretch and warm up the muscles in your feet, ankles, legs, and back. If you have arthritis in your elbow joints, walk while swinging your arms at the elbow.

SWIMMING

Swimming can help people with every kind of OA. You can make a real splash with your progress by diving into a swimming routine. There are several options for achieving and maintaining fitness for water lovers.

Chances are you don't have a pool in your backyard, but there are surely health clubs, YMCAs or YWCAs, hospitals, and municipal facilities nearby that do. As mentioned earlier, you'll need to find out what times are available for free swimming, as well as the temperature of the water, and any classes available.

If laps are what you're after, take your time getting acquainted with the water, and be sure you breathe efficiently. Consult an instructor to help get your form down, and if he or she is qualified, ask for specific exercises to help work the joints that most trouble you. Use a snorkel if the pain in your neck prevents you from turning your head to the side. Use a kickboard if you don't have the upper body strength you need to carry you confidently. And check out an inner tube for around your waist if you want to remain stationary, but still work those hips and knees. There are other devices that can help you reach your goals. Just shop around a little and you'll be amazed at what's out there.

And even though some people don't think it's as good a workout as walking, there's still evidence that those who swim have thicker bones than people who don't exercise at all. That says a lot for the sport, but what will really speak to you is how much better you feel after doing water sports, and how quickly they can improve your flexibility and decrease pain. Many people with OA who give themselves to water activities say they work more thoroughly and create

**DON'T
NEGLECT
YOUR REST**

It's as important to
rest your joints
between sessions
as it is to do your
workout. What's
more, it's critical
to take a break
during your rou-
tine if a joint starts
to hurt. To ward
off pain in elbows
or knees, exercise
with a neoprene
or elastic brace or
tape to stabilize
the joint. A
wedged insole
with a five- or ten-
degree angle can
also help with mild
or moderate pain
in the knees. If
you have arthritis
in the neck, shoul-
der or back, use a
collar, sling, or
corset to relieve
the pressure and
subsequent pain.
Any activity that
causes pain that
lasts for more than
two hours should
not be repeated.[3]

results faster than any other form of exercise.
Because of water's natural buoyancy and the low-
impact nature of water activity, swimming is ideal
for anyone with OA or who is overweight.

WATER AEROBICS

Laps are wonderful, but so are water aerobics
classes, or even self-directed sessions of running or
walking in the pool. Your routine can be as simple
as walking back and forth between the shallow ends
of the pool, or running as far as you can until you
reach the deep end, then breaking out into a free-
style, sidestroke, or backstroke swim. No matter
what you do in the water, it's easier than on land
since there is little pressure against your joints and
muscles.

If you're new to water aerobics and somewhat
tenuous about it, start slowly by entering the shallow end and doing the Arthritis Cure Fitness Plan
warm-up/cool down exercises with your lower
extremities. You'll probably find it very enjoyable,
and before you know it, you'll be going deeper and
doing the Arthritis Cure Fitness Plan warm-up/cool
down exercises for your upper body. Try going up to
your neck and freely walk, run, or dance around the
pool. Your time in the water doesn't have to be
structured, but like all aerobics, it does need to be
constant in order to get your heart rate up and
strengthen the muscles.

Start slowly and at a pace that suits you. But
shoot for a good thirty-five–minute routine three
days a week. You may have to work up to that over
a month, maybe even a year.

BICYCLING

Getting on a bike and cruising around is plain old fun. You cover more ground than walking, and it provides great opportunities to strengthen leg muscles and lubricate the knees.

If you're attracted to biking as your cardio workout but don't have one, consider buying a new one. Mountain bikes have fat, stubby tires that are less inclined to go flat from sharp rocks or road debris, and provide more stability than bikes with skinny tires. You can get a good one for about $200, but there are models that cost less. Also, look for used bikes for sale in your local paper; you can usually find a good bargain.

The multiple-gearing system on new bikes is a bit more complicated. Ask the sales clerk for a detailed explanation of how they work, then play around with them on flat land. You'll quickly dis-

STREET-SMART BIKING

There are some basic rules of riding that can save you everything from big scares to hospital bills.

First, helmets are a necessity. Seventy-five percent of bicycle-related fatalities are due to head injuries. Wearing a helmet would have increased the survival rate by 85 percent. Common sense, or street smarts, is all you need to realize the importance of strapping on a good helmet.

Other tidbits:

- Ride in the same direction as traffic.
- Talk with an expert or qualified bicyclist about how to safely control your brakes and manage your gears.
- Honor traffic signals and signs.
- Give the right of way to cars.
- If you ride at night, get a headlight and reflective clothing. (Riding at night is dangerous, so do it only if you have to, otherwise, it's not worth the risk.)
- Use rear-view mirrors.
- Avoid dangerous terrain.
- Save the Walkman for indoor activities.
- Learn to change a flat tire, or wear a cellular phone to call someone if you get a flat.

cover how the gears enable you to pedal really fast and hard on flat land, and fairly easily up steep inclines. Pretty soon, you'll be planning a trip to the mountains so you can conquer a few hills and race down the opposite side.

Helmets are a must. Don't skimp on quality—these things can save you from injury and possibly your life. Ask a knowledgeable salesclerk about the best brand, and ensure a proper fit.

ANKLE INJURIES AND HOW TO TREAT THEM

The best way to treat an ankle injury is to avoid getting one in the first place. Prevention includes supportive shoes, proper posture, strengthening leg muscles, and carrying your weight squarely over your hips and feet.

Sprains typically occur when the foot twists inward and the outside ligament is then stretched or torn. Fewer sprains involve an outward twist of the foot that then pulls or tears the inside ligaments.

There are three kinds of sprains:

FIRST DEGREE. In this case a ligament is slightly torn with accompanying mild pain, tenderness and swelling. You may be unable to place your full weight on the foot, but this type of sprain won't radically disrupt your lifestyle. Even so, it can take up to six weeks to heal completely.

SECOND DEGREE. This one is a bit more serious, and the sensations that go along with it prove it. You will feel a pop or snap, followed by swelling, tenderness, and, within a few days, bruising. Here, you'd find it hard to walk and would have to recuperate for up to eight weeks.

THIRD DEGREE. This is a bad one where the joint slips out of place then back in upon impact. You probably won't be able to walk, and the swelling, tenderness, and pain may indicate that corrective surgery is necessary. Recovery can take as long as twelve weeks.

Regardless of what you diagnose for yourself, you should contact a doctor immediately after an ankle injury to get X rays and rule out a fracture. But before you get to the doctor, you can treat the injury with RICE, or Rest, Ice, Compression, and Elevation. Get ice on it as soon as possible.

Once you rule out a fracture, keep the ankle iced for ten-to thirty-minute intervals. Continue to ice it on and off for seventy-two hours, compress the ankle with an ace bandage, and keep your foot elevated above your hip.

Don't resume exercise until the injury is completely healed; you can do more damage, and extend your recovery time by worsening the injury.

Water cages, as they're called, and lightweight water bottles that fit snugly into the cages are also a must. They are typically right under the handlebars for easy access while you're riding.

Other equipment is available that can help your ride be more efficient or comfortable. There are special handlebars for people with back problems. They are designed so that riders don't need to lean so far forward. It makes "touring" more comfortable. Biking gloves cushion your palms from the weight you'll distribute as you lean on the handlebars. Biking shorts are specially padded in the crotch to ease the stress there. And you can attach toe clips to the pedals so you use energy more efficiently while pumping. Bike racks can also be purchased so you don't have to ride your bike through traffic to get to the less congested bike path or road of choice. (These accoutrements are helpful but not *crucial* to get a good *workout*.)

Once you've got the perfect bike and bought whatever gear you're after, it might be a good idea to have a friend nearby the first time you saddle up. If you're feeling unstable, don't take a chance and go it alone.

As always, take it easy your first day out. If one lap around the block is all you can manage, that's fine. On the other hand, if you're feeling pretty comfortable, try for two or three. Remember, if you're not doing a loop, you'll have to turn around and go back as far as you've come. So don't exhaust yourself before turning around.

As your body grows accustomed to the routine, you can work your way to that thirty-minute goal, two to three days a week.

AEROBICS

Just about any fitness center or gym in the country offers a grand array of aerobics classes from jazzercise to step classes to water aerobics. Use common sense and think about your special needs. If you're attracted to a jazzercise class, but have a difficult time moving at the hips, it might be wise to start with a less active class.

The first thing to do is to contact the instructor of the class you want to take. And, of course, it doesn't have to be one offered at a gym. Aerobic activity covers anything that makes you move enough to increase your heart rate for a sustained period of time. So if you find out about a dance class—whether it's ballroom, jitterbugging, country line dancing, or modern or folk dancing—they qualify as aerobics classes, too. In any case, since you have special needs, it's important to speak to the instructor to find out exactly how strenuous the class is and determine if you can do it comfortably. If you think you can, call your doctor and make sure there's no objection from that end.

Aerobics classes can be low-impact (which is probably where you want to start), moderately difficult, or high-impact for advanced exercisers. Some classes can involve nonstop movement for up to sixty minutes, and that can be hard even if you don't have OA. It might be wise to observe a class first, then determine if it's what you want.

And part of determining that is to see if it looks like fun and like something you *want* to do.

If you're not sure about how the class could affect you, remember that you can do it at your own pace. You can take breaks even when others keep on moving. You can (and should) take water breaks. You can tailor the workout to meet your needs as long as you've discussed it with the instructor beforehand.

The beauty of aerobics classes is that they can bring some real fun into your exercise routine. They expose you to a group of people who can extend into your social circle. They promote flexibility, strengthening, and cardiovascular activities, all of which you need to loosen joints and pump up muscles. And some people say that dance classes make them feel twenty years younger. All that adds up to a good time with spirits lifted, and plenty of good movement for your body.

Don't forget to wear good aerobic shoes for classes at the gym, and if you're out dancing, be sure the shoes you wear are appropriate. High heels are discouraged. Visit your local shoe store and check out the cushioned-soled shoes with a more formal appearance. There are ways to look good and be comfortable (and safe), too.

You have to be the judge of your own capabilities, so work with your body, enjoy yourself, and aim for that thirty-minute marker. Although most classes will have a warm-up period and a very short cool down, you will want to maintain your Arthritis Cure Fitness Plan warm-up/cool down and stretches to maximize the benefit of your cardiovascular activity, and stay flexible for the next class.

Aerobics classes can be beneficial to people with OA in any part of their body. If it's in your knees, however, be wise about what types of movements you make so that you don't jar or twist them unnecessarily. And if your fingers feel the pain, be sure your dancing partners are sensitive and don't clutch them too tightly.

There are also classes designed especially for people with OA. Call the local chapter of the Arthritis Foundation and see if they know of any. Or, call the nearest hospital or a physical therapist.

THE NEXT STEP

Now that you've integrated these four steps into your life, you are now a bona fide exercise expert—well, at least you are on your way. Here are some suggestions to modify your workout:

Increase your workout time: If possible, add in regular increments, time to your cardio workouts—from thirty minutes to thirty-five to forty, etc.

THE QUAD QUANDARY

How could weak muscles in the upper leg lead to arthritis in the knee? Consider that the quadriceps, a set of four muscles in the front part of the leg above the knee, provide strength to the knee joint and influence how you extend your leg when you walk. Those with strong quadriceps are able to control how hard their feet hit the ground when they walk, reducing impact stress on knee joints. People with weak quadriceps, on the other hand, lack that leg control and tend to put their feet down too forcefully when they take steps. That puts unnecessary stress on the knee, which could lead to a breakdown of knee joint cartilage that cushions the knee bones. As the cartilage deteriorates, the bones start rubbing together, causing the loss of joint alignment that is one of the hallmarks of OA.

—*Tufts University Health & Nutrition Letter, Oct. 1997.*

	MON.	TUES.	WED.	THURS.	FRI.	SAT.	SUN.
WEEK I	AM: warm-up/cool down PM: warm-up/cool down	AM: warm-up/cool down PM: warm-up/cool down	AM: warm-up/cool down PM: warm-up/cool down	AM: warm-up/cool down PM: warm-up/cool down	AM: warm-up/cool down PM: warm-up/cool down	Recreation	Rest
WEEK II	AM: warm-up/cool down; stretching PM: warm-up/cool down	AM: warm-up/cool down; stretching PM: warm-up/cool down	AM: warm-up/cool down; stretching PM: warm-up/cool down	AM: warm-up/cool down; stretching PM: warm-up/cool down	AM: warm-up/cool down; stretching PM: warm-up/cool down	Yoga	Rest
WEEK III	WHOLE WORKOUT ANYTIME: warm-up/cool down; stretching; muscle strengthening; warm-up/cool down	AM: warm-up/cool down; stretching PM: warm-up/cool down	WHOLE WORKOUT ANYTIME: warm-up/cool down; stretching; muscle strengthening; warm-up/cool down	AM: warm-up/cool down; stretching PM: warm-up/cool down	WHOLE WORKOUT ANYTIME: warm-up/cool down; stretching; muscle strengthening; warm-up/cool down	Recreation	Rest
WEEK IV	WHOLE WORKOUT ANYTIME: warm-up/cool down; stretching; muscle strengthening; warm-up/cool down	WHOLE WORKOUT ANYTIME: warm-up/cool down; stretching; cardio workout (at least 30 min.); warm-up/cool down	WHOLE WORKOUT ANYTIME: warm-up/cool down; stretching; muscle strengthening; warm-up/cool down	WHOLE WORKOUT ANYTIME: warm-up/cool down; stretching; cardio workout (at least 30 min.); warm-up/cool down	WHOLE WORKOUT ANYTIME: warm-up/cool down; stretching; muscle strengthening; warm-up/cool down	Yoga	Rest

- Consult a personal trainer and fitness expert and add new musc strengthening moves to your workout.
- During muscle strengthening moves increase your weight/resis ance and/or number of repetitions.
- Cross-train, meaning incorporate different workouts into yo weekly routine. Try new things.

MODIFICATIONS AND SPECIAL CONCERNS

o successfully maintain your new routine, you must be mindful of our overall fitness needs. Look at what you've set up for yourself, valuate what is and is not going well for you, and rework the pro-ram so it works *for* you rather than *against* you. If your muscles never top aching, you're probably pushing too hard—lighten up a bit. If ou know you could push harder than you have been, then do it. Reap ne benefits and exercise yourself into a new level of wellness.

And for those of you with other physical concerns such as high lood pressure, diabetes, low blood sugar, or hyper- or hypothyroid, e sure to consult with your physician about how your new routine night impact these conditions, and how you can most effectively nanage your overall health. Don't take chances with your health.

CHAPTER SIX

Yoga and Mind/Body Techniques

"I honestly think there is no limit to what breathwork can accomplish—not only in areas of physical and emotional health, but also as a way of increasing mindfulness and spiritual awareness."

—DR. ANDREW WEIL

Yoga, *qigong*, and *tai chi* may sound like Chinese to you, but for millions of people across America, they're household words—and activities. These practices are as ancient as they are beneficial. Part of what's beneficial is that they're more meditative than fast-moving workouts. That means they generally employ very slow, methodic, and gentle movements, as well as a focus on consciousness. Each of these techniques contain at least a three-pronged approach to health: improved muscle flexibility, strength, and tone; proper breathing; and relaxation, which may include creative visualization or other closed-eye exercises. This may sound strange, but studies show they're good medicine for people with OA. In fact, Dr. Dean Ornish, author of *Dr. Dean Ornish's Program for Reversing Heart Disease*, recommends yoga to help people prevent or reverse heart disease. Hospitals around the country have now integrated yoga into their programs for treating chronic pain, stress-related medical disorders, and patients who have had heart attacks.[1]

PROOF POSITIVE BENEFITS OF YOGA

Suza Francina, a certified Iyengar Yoga instructor with more than twenty years of experience in the field of yoga and exercise therapy and the director of the Ojai Yoga Center in Ojai, California, says "Arthritis need not mean a prognosis of inevitable disability. By practicing (yoga) consistently, every day, you can reduce pain, build your strength and live with health and renewed energy.... Yoga is an ideal form of exercise because its movements are fluid and adaptable. Moreover, students progress gradually, beginning with simple stretches and strengthening poses, and advancing to more difficult postures only as they become stronger and more flexible. For those with moderate and good levels of balance and flexibility, you can begin yoga with gentle movements sitting in a chair or lying on the floor, if necessary. Simple 'one-joint' movements will gently loosen your joints and relax your muscles. These therapeutic yoga-based movements also improve your breathing and help relieve physical and emotional tension."

YOGA STRETCHING POSITIONS

When doing yoga avoid extending your limbs abruptly or in unnatural directions. Also, be careful not to hold a single position for too long—not to the point where your body feels unhealthy strain or stiffens up from leaving muscles in a static position too long.

In the following exercises, hands and wrists should not be placed in any position that accentuates or encourages deformity. Every movement should be designed to move the hand back toward normal.

Namaste (prayer) Position: Sit or stand and press your palms together in prayer position. This position helps to stretch the muscles in the hand and straighten the fingers. If you have arthritic wrists or carpal tunnel syndrome, practice Namaste with forearms touching.

Gently press the palms and fingers of both hands together. As you breathe smoothly and evenly, encourage the fingers to move toward the thumb side of the hand. Hold for several breaths. Release the pressure but keep the hands together for a few more breaths. Then repeat the effort three or four times.

Gently, firmly, and evenly press the palms together. Smoothly open the fingers and spread them as wide as possible. Try to spread them evenly, moving them more and more toward the thumb side of the hand. Hold and stretch for a few breaths. Release and repeat.

Firmly and evenly press the palms together, especially the parts of the palm at the base of each finger. Stretch the fingers backward, away from each other, gradually increasing the V-shaped space between them. Again, encourage the fingers to move toward the thumb side of the hand. Encourage your fingers to stretch for three or four more breaths. Release and repeat three or four more times.

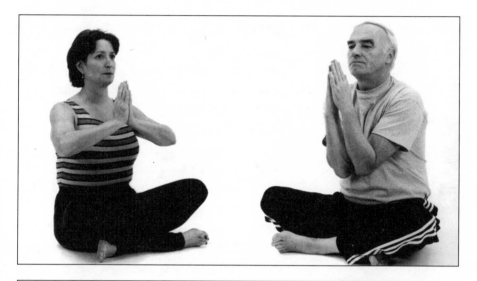

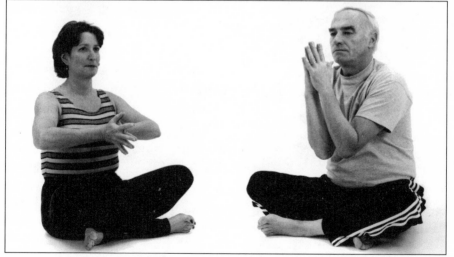

To avoid pulled muscles, overstretching, and joint strain, never force or rush your body into a yoga position. Use straps and belts, instead, to help you achieve a healthier, more balanced stretch. If you cannot clasp your hands together, use a strap as a bridge between your two hands. This shoulder rotator exercise is one of the most basic corrective poses for removing stiffness from the shoulder joints: Stand (or sit) in your best, tallest posture. Pause for a moment to observe your breath. Allow yourself to smile. This will naturally relax your jaw and face muscles.

Behind the Back Clasp: Stretch your right arm straight up over your head and then bend your elbow so that your palm touches your back between the shoulder blades. Reach across with your left hand to move your elbow closer to your head.

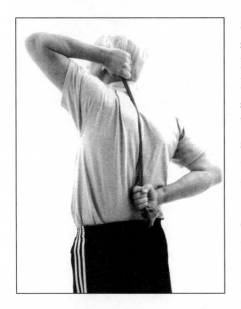

Release your left hand from your right elbow and bring your left arm straight back behind your body. Bend the left elbow, placing your hand in the middle of your back above your waist, palm out. Without distorting your posture or straining, try to clasp your hands together. If this is not possible, try using a towel or elastic band.

If your fingers just barely touch, or if there is a big space between your hands, hold a strap or sock in your right hand and gradually work your hands together. Stretch up through the top elbow and down through the bottom elbow. Keep your head centered, face relaxed. Hold at least half a minute. Repeat on the right side. If you have a more flexible side repeat or hold longer on the tighter side.

Triangle Pose at Wall: Make sure you have at least six feet of empty wall space. To improve posture, spend a few minutes every day standing "tall" with your back against the wall. If you tend to stoop forward, stretch your shoulders back and stand against the wall several times a day.

Stand tall with your posture open, shoulders relaxed away from your ears, near the wall. Spread your feet about three and a half to four feet apart (depending on the length of your legs), keeping your feet in line, facing forward, heels close to the wall.

Breathe normally. Anchor and root your feet to the earth by pressing the soles of your feet deep into the floor. Activate your legs by pulling up the thigh muscles. Allow your body to become taller and taller, stretching your spine upward. Raise your arms to shoulder level, palms facing down, and stretch out through your fingertips. Feel the center of your body expand and open.

When you feel stable and centered in this position, turn the left foot about fifteen degrees in, and the right foot ninety degrees out. Line up the right heel directly in line with the center of the left arch.

THE RIPPLE EFFECT

Yoga is perhaps the most popular of these mind/body exercises. Yoga classes are offered through yoga centers, hospitals, gyms, dance studios, and colleges, or by private instruction. There are also books and videotapes with detailed instruction that you can do at home. Like the other disciplines, yoga addresses "the whole person" and can be of help to people with a broad range of medical problems. The word itself, "yoga" is Sanskrit and means "to unite, to make whole."[2] So, if you're battling with more than OA, yoga might be an excellent resource.

Stretching is an integral part of what makes up yoga. But the stretches you'll do in these classes go beyond what you've ever done before—not in terms of *stressing* the muscles—but by taking on postures or positions that stretch several muscles at once. And according to the philosophy behind yoga, these positions open up the lines of energy that flow through our bodies, thus enabling more energy to blocked areas (such as your arthritic joints). The theory is that when energy flows to those areas, there's a greater opportunity for healing. It's almost certain you'll experience greater movement, strength, and inner peace if you utilize this wonderful approach to health.

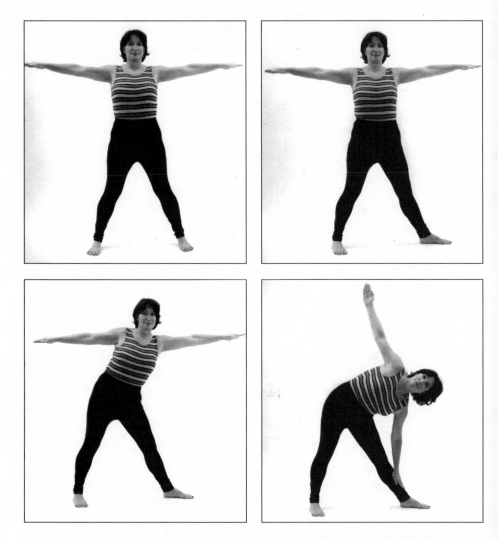

Inhale, and on exhalation, stretch to the right from the hip joint, so your torso bends sideways as a unit toward your right leg. In the beginning, you may need to place your right hand on your leg, a chair, or block. Extend your left arm up in line with the right arm, palm facing forward. If you feel unusual strain in your shoulder, try placing your left hand on your hip.

Stay in the pose for several breaths, keeping your legs active, shoulders and neck relaxed. Come out of the pose on an inhalation, keeping your body close to the wall. Turn your feet to face forward. Relax back into the wall and pause for a moment to feel the effects of the pose. Repeat on the other side.

Downward Facing Dog Pose from the Floor (For Advanced Exercisers Only): Kneel on all fours on a nonslippery floor, so that your hands do not slide. Position your knees slightly behind your hips, toes curled under, your feet and knees hip-width (about eighteen inches) apart. Place your hands slightly in front of your shoulders, shoulder-distance apart. Spread all ten fingers wide apart and press both hands down onto the floor.

On an exhale, straighten your knees and lift your bottom toward the ceiling so that your body forms a high upside-down V or pyramid shape. Raise your heels high off the floor and try to lift your bottom higher and higher. Press your hands deep into the floor as if you are pushing the floor away from you. After stretching for a few breaths with your heels lifted, try pressing your heels down toward the floor.

FROM CAN'T TO CAN

Unlike other forms of physical exercise, yoga has something for everyone. No one is excluded. People with chronic disease and disabilities face "can't" at every turn in their lives: they can't play golf, can't play tennis, can't run, can't overexert themselves, can't walk without canes, some can't walk at all. But everyone can do yoga. In yoga, there are no can'ts. Yoga can be modified and adapted to suit the needs of everyone.

—Lorna Bell, R.N.
Gentle Yoga for People with Arthritis, Stroke Damage, Multiple Sclerosis and in Wheelchairs

These slow, deliberate stretches, and the proper breathing that you'll learn while doing them, can be done at your own individual pace. You get to take yourself to the limits of your own body without stressing or straining yourself. Of course, you might be seated next to someone who can touch her nose to her knees without any difficulty. But that's *her* flexibility, not yours. The great news about yoga is that it will help everyone at any level of strength or flexibility. As long as you don't push yourself too hard, or set up rules of competition within your own head, then you can reap the benefits of this wonderful exercise no matter what shape you're in.

Clearly, yoga could help no matter where your joints are affected by OA. But if your fingers are the target, take note: Recent studies show that yoga designed especially for people with OA of the hands reduced pain and increased finger range of motion after only eight sessions. The movements helped with problematic posture and alignment, too. [3]

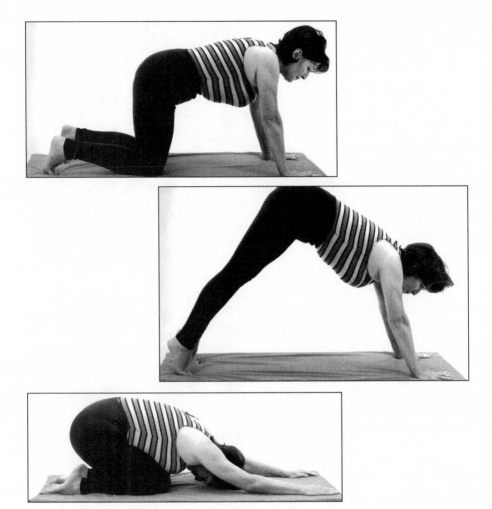

Breathe smoothly, naturally. Keep your face and neck relaxed and soft. Imagine roots pulling your hands and feet into the earth while the top of your buttocks—your tailbone—extends toward the sky. Release, come back to kneeling on all fours. Slowly lower your bottom back toward your heels and lower your torso and forehead to the floor.

A common complaint in this pose is pressure on the wrists. If your wrists are extremely sensitive, place a folded mat (or folded blanket on the mat to keep it from slipping) under the heel of your hands, so that the wrist part of your hand is slightly elevated and supported by the extra cushioning.

Do not stay in the pose if your back hurts, if you feel unusual pressure in the head, or dizziness, or if your wrists and shoulders ache.

Lying-Down Leg Stretch with a Strap: A strap, towel, or soft belt around your feet while lying on the floor helps your spine to remain long and stable. Using a strap allows you to gradually stretch and lengthen stiff leg muscles without straining your back.

Lie on your back with your knees bent, feet flat on the floor. If your head tilts back with your chin higher than your forehead, place a folded blanket under your head and neck. Check to see that your upper body is in line with your legs. Allow your back to relax into the floor.

Bend your right knee in toward your chest and wrap a strap, towel, soft belt or necktie around the ball of your foot. Hold the strap with your right hand.

Slowly straighten your right leg and stretch your toes toward your face. Walk your hand higher up the strap toward your foot till your arm is straight. Keep your shoulders and the rest of your back relaxed on the floor.

If your right hand is quite far away from your foot, keep your left knee bent. If you find it easy to hold your big toe, or if your right hand is high up the strap close to your foot, you can deepen the stretch

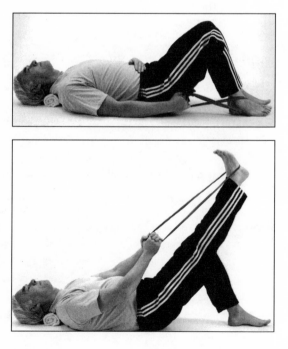

by practicing this pose with the bottom leg straight, extending through both heels. Stretch your toes toward your face to lengthen your calves and Achilles tendons.

Smile and allow your face muscles to relax. Let your breath flow freely, stretching deeper as you exhale. Hold the strap firmly without creating tension in your hand. Enjoy the feeling of the back of your leg lengthening. Hold for about half a minute, longer as you learn to relax and cooperate with the pose. Repeat on the opposite side. If you are practicing with both legs straight, it is helpful to extend the lower heel into a wall.

As always, approach yoga with an awareness of your own needs and limitations, and monitor your progress daily. If your body feels better after you do it, you probably did it right. If it feels bad, you did something wrong. Talk with a qualified instructor or a physical therapist who knows about yoga techniques, and get to the root of the problem before it gets to you.

When you consult your doctor about doing yoga, don't be sur-

HOPE FOR KNEES AND HIPS

"I might be in a wheelchair or much worse, if not for yoga," said one seventy-eight-year-old student who has been attending class two or three times a week for the last four years. Diagnosed with OA in her knees two years before she started yoga, she had pain in her left hip, pins in her right hip (which was without pain), a left leg shorter than her right, and a hearing problem that affected her balance. When she first started yoga, she had to sit down or hold onto a support to do anything that required standing on one foot.

This student first started standing poses with the help of a wall, chair, and wall ropes. She practiced at home using a kitchen counter or table. As her balance improved, she began to practice the poses in the middle of the room....Three years later, she is able to practice with her feet wide apart and her balance and alignment are beautiful. She enjoys staying in the poses. In class, she is usually the last person to come out of the pose.

—*The New Yoga for People Over 50*, Suza Francina

prised if he or she is hesitant or doesn't really know how it could be of benefit to you. Many "mainstream" doctors don't consider options outside their own specialty. If you decide to pursue it and it's of benefit to you, call your doctor and report the good news. Then he or she may be more open to the next patient asking about alternative treatments.

Qigong and tai chi are other methodologies that could be of benefit to your condition. There are books available that teach these techniques directly to people with arthritis. Call your local bookstore or ask a health-care practitioner whose studies may include these techniques.

CHAPTER SEVEN

Fitness & Nutrition: Evaluating Your Eating Habits

"To eat is human, to digest is divine."

—Mark Twain

OPEN YOUR REFRIGERATOR AND take a quick inventory. Do the same for the items in your pantry. Are your shelves filled with "empty-calorie" fillers—sweets, chips, and soda, or whole, healthy, unprocessed foods? What do you reach for when you want a quick pick-me-up? Are you aware of the emotions that cause you to eat? Do you know which are your "comfort foods"? Do you frequently give in to cravings even when you're not really hungry? Notice, too, the atmosphere in which you normally dine. Do you create a special place for your meals so that you can relax and enjoy your food (doing this facilitates digestion and enhances nutrient absorption)? Or, do you eat on the run, at your desk, in the car, in front of the television while watching the evening news? Are you a "grazer," picking at food all day, or do you take time to plan your meals carefully?

An essential part of the Arthritis Cure Fitness Plan is making sure your food choices support your ultimate goal of health and well-being. Your food choices can either help to alleviate or to aggravate your OA condition. It is important to know those foods that actually trigger pain and those that promote good health.

Being aware of your nutritional needs is as crucial to your extended health and happiness as is your commitment to exercise and fitness. And meeting those challenges with a clear, open mind will secure your success even more. It may require making a major lifestyle change. But there will be "bonus" benefits to your new diet. You'll not only see improvements in your physical body, but it's likely you'll also notice improvement in your mood and mental outlook. If you have other health concerns, such as high cholesterol, high blood pressure, or diabetes, a revised diet will register positive effects there, too.

HOW YOU RELATE TO FOOD

The majority of people with OA are overweight. And most are not overweight due to medical problems, but rather due to unawareness of the effects of eating certain foods and to their poor relationship with food.

Answer the following questions to find out your relationship with food:

1. Do you eat when you're emotional? If so, what are the dominant emotions that drive you to eat (i.e. anger, depression, resentment, elation, jealousy, powerlessness, excitement)?

TREAT YOUR OA— AND ALSO ENJOY...

A STRONGER IMMUNE SYSTEM:

When you eat foods that nourish and strengthen your body, you'll not only feel better physically, you'll also have an improved outlook on life. In turn, your immune system will become stronger and better able to address the challenges caused by OA.

LOWERING OF HIGH BLOOD PRESSURE:

Obesity and diets heavy in salt, alcohol, and fatty or sugary foods can bring on or aggravate high blood pressure and cholesterol, or hypertension. Those types of foods also increase the risk of stroke and heart disease. The OA-friendly diet combats all those conditions.

BETTER MANAGEMENT OF DIABETES:

The most common form of diabetes is *diabetes mellitus*, and it results from a deficiency of insulin in the body. It often runs in families. Diet plays a critical role in the treatment of diabetes, and eating whole, unprocessed foods and avoiding salt, sugar, and other empty calories will help the diabetes as well as the joints.

2. What are the foods that you crave when you're emotional?
3. Do you find comfort in those foods, or do they actually make you feel worse after you've eaten them?
4. Do you often eat when you're not hungry?
5. Could you call yourself "addicted" to a specific food or foods?
6. What is it about food that makes you want it? Does it fill up an emptiness inside you? Is it the taste that satisfies you? Does it remind you of something from the past that makes you feel good?
7. If you could take control of your eating habits, when would you eat? How much? What kinds of foods?
8. Are you willing to give up eating certain foods (most of the time) that you love? If so, why? If not, why not?
9. Do you like to cook? If so, what do you like about it? If not, what do you dislike about it?
10. If you had a choice of eating only one food for the rest of your life, what would it be?

Your relationship with food may have a powerful hold over you, and simply telling yourself to change your habits may not be enough to carry out a lasting change. You might need to heal a past pain, face a current one, or give up an insatiable need for instant gratification that's rooted in something you may not even understand.

Very often overeating, binge eating, or simply eating "all the time" is a way for people to "eat away" or avoid their problems. Maybe you are on bad terms with your spouse or children, depressed about experiencing so much pain, or unhappy with yourself or your life situation. Or maybe your car didn't start this morning. Problems can be big or small, but turning to food is a typical "answer" for many people.

If you suspect this may be the case for you, consider seeking professional help. There are counselors and therapists who specialize in eating disorders. You may not consider yourself as someone with an eating disorder, but keep in mind that if you are more than twenty

EAT IT AND JOT IT

Consider keeping a journal and recording your daily food intake. It can be used to make sure you are getting a well-balanced diet and to show how emotions play into your eating habits. Use it to help reach your goals. Try it for at least two months, and decide if you have enough awareness and have established good enough eating habits so that you no longer need it. Don't worry about fat content or calories (unless, of course, you want to). Just write down:

1. What time it is.
2. What you ate.
3. How much you ate (i.e. small portion, medium portion, one apple, three servings of mashed potatoes, etc.)
4. How you felt when you were eating.
5. How you felt after you ate.

pounds overweight, and have been for more than a year, you probably turn to foods in unhealthy ways. Professional help or even a visit to your local chapter of Overeater's Anonymous could dramatically change your life—for the better.

AN HONEST LOOK AT FOOD

Just *how* fattening and caloric *are* some of your favorite foods? Let's take a look at some old favorites and compare them to what will hopefully become some new favorites:

Old favorite—breakfast (These figures are approximate and may vary according to brand)[1]:

Food	Amount	Fat Grams	Calories	% Fat Calories
6" buttermilk pancake (no butter or syrup)	3	15	490	28%
Butter	1 tbsp.	7	70	100%
Maple syrup	1/4 cup	0	210	0
Italian Pork Sausage	3 oz.	21	268	71%
White bread toast	2 slices	2	70	26%
Butter (for toast)	1 tbsp.	7	70	100%
Orange Juice	8 oz.	0	130	0
Coffee	6 oz.	0	4	0
Half & Half	2 tbsp.	3	40	68%
Sugar	1 tsp.	0	15	0

This old favorite breakfast adds up to:

55 grams of fat (that's the approximately *total* amount you should be consuming in one day!)

1367 calories (if you estimate a 2000 calorie

a day limit, you'll likely go over the limit for the day).

Now, let's compare this to a new favorite breakfast:

Food	Amount	Fat Grams	Calories	% Fat Calories
Cantaloupe	1 cup	< 1	57	8%
Raisin Bran Cereal	1 cup	1	170	5%
Skim milk	1/2 cup	0	46	0
Banana	1 medium	0	110	0
Wheat bread toast	2 slices	3	90	15%
Apple jelly	2 tsp.	0	30	0
Coffee	6 oz.	0	4	0
Mocha mix nondairy creamer	2 tbsp.	4	40	100%
Orange Juice	8 oz.	0	130	0

Here's what this healthy breakfast adds up to:

Approximately 9 grams of fat and 677 calories. Big difference.

Here are some other old favorite foods that may be making your

SETTING GOALS

Write down five goals you'd like to reach as a member of the Arthritis Cure Fitness Team. Examples might include:

1. I want to relieve the pain in my joints.
2. I want to lose fifty pounds so that my constant weight is one hundred fifty pounds.
3. I want to meet other people who are committed to health and fitness so I can find inspiration in knowing them.
4. I want to improve my sex life by feeling more attractive and experiencing the feeling of vitality.
5. I want to go on vacation with my spouse for a long-overdue second honeymoon.

Once you've recorded your goals, then look at them and decide realistically when you think they can be achieved. Write how many weeks or months you think it will take, and a "goal date" for having attained them.

The goals may change; and once you've achieved one goal, replace it with another. As you cross the old ones off your list, reward yourself—flowers, a double feature, a weekend trip to a spa, a new bike.

OA condition worse. Pay close attention to the fat content, and be aware that the amounts listed may be less than what you consume at an average meal.

Food	Amount	Fat Grams	Calories	% Fat Calories
Chocolate croissant	1	23	370	56%
McDonalds Quarter Pounder with cheese	1	30	530	51%
McDonalds large French Fries	1 order	22	450	44%
Taco Bell Chicken Supreme Burrito	1	23	520	40%
12" cheese, sausage, & mushroom pizza	2/5 pizza	32	640	90%
Baskin & Robbins French vanilla ice cream	1/2 cup	11	160	62%
Swanson Hungry Man Beef & Broccoli frozen dinner	1 dinner	16	500	29%
Pepperidge Farm Chesapeake chocolate chunk pecan cookie	2 cookies	16	280	100%
Boston Cream Pie	1/6 cake	12	290	37%

HEALTHY EATING: THE BASICS

Eating is a very personal experience. For some people, it feels like the only aspect of life over which they have control. Which is true—you do have control over what you eat. As you discover your relationship with food, take a new kind of control and begin eating new foods, healthier foods, less fattening foods. If you follow the tips below for one week, you will, by week's end, realize that the choices don't have to be different, and that they can afford you delicious flavors, and a satisfied appetite.

1. Try not to eat when you're angry or upset (not even when you're overly excited). Don't use food as solace for your emotions.
2. Whenever there's an option, try to buy only nonfat or low-fat

items, such as milk, salad dressings, sweets, and other foods. But remember, several nonfat or low-fat foods (especially desserts) typically contain plenty of sugar and calories which, if you're not exercising regularly, can turn to fat within your body.

3. Avoid fast-food restaurants *whenever possible.* This may seem impossible, but when you're on the go and need a quick bite, remember, there are other options. Instead of heading for the drive-through of the local (high-fat) burger joint, go to a grocery store or deli instead. Select healthy sandwiches with mustard or nonfat mayonnaise. If you're travelling and don't know where a market is located, at least go for the fast-food places with low-fat alternatives, such as Subway. If the only choices before you are McDonalds or Burger King, then order a salad without the dressing, or a grilled chicken sandwich, again, without condiments. It may take a little while to rearrange your habits, but once you start thinking about it, you'll find that it's fun to be creative and find ways around eating high-fat foods.

4. Fill up on fruits and vegetables. Whether for breakfast, lunch, dinner, or in between snacks, these foods are the way to go. Splurge and try exotic fruits you may have avoided like mangos, papayas, kiwis, and melons. They're all delicious, sweet, and good for you. Exotic vegetables are fun too, like plantains, various squashes, and different types of mushrooms. The old standards are fine, too. Keep bite-sized carrots, celery, broccoli, and green and red peppers on hand to satisfy the need to crunch. You can even jazz them up with a nonfat dip. Rely on these healthy alternatives especially when craving a snack, and avoid those cookies, crackers, and chips.

5. Limit your portions. Try not to eat more than six ounces (even try four ounces) of meat, poultry, or fish, at a sitting. Pile on vegetables or fruits to compensate for the smaller portion of meat. Also use a smaller plate, and stop after one helping.

6. Nix the oil and butter. Again, it takes a while to break old

habits, but you don't have to cook everything in butter or oil. Use nonstick cookware or nonstick spray if you need to, and bake, poach, or boil your foods. Once the foods are cooked, don't reach for the butter. You may realize how you've been missing the true flavors of the foods that were being masked by the butter. If you want a little zest, add vinegar, lemon, or spices—especially cardamom, curry, garlic, cinnamon, and ginger—all of which reduce inflammation.

7. Eat slowly and ritualistically. Turn off the television. Sit down with your spouse or make a special place for yourself at the table. Maybe place some flowers near you on the table or play some dinner music. Take time to make eating an activity that you relish and enjoy. Chew deliberately. Taste it. Explore the flavors. Eating can be a healthy *and* comforting experience, one that is indeed in your control.

Once you've broken the trail to eating more healthfully, you'll want to learn more about how you can support yourself nutritionally. There are hundreds of great books on the market about smart eating, but our favorite is *The Arthritis Cure Cookbook,* our companion guide to this book. The book provides tips for how to get excited about cooking, how to make cooking easier, and it's filled with arthritis-smart recipes (yes, some of them even include small amounts of butter and sugar!) that will satisfy even the pickiest eater. In it, you'll learn all kinds of valuable things, for example: Green vegetables contain omega three fatty acids that block the chemicals that cause inflammation. Fish and marine vegetables also contain an ingredient that do the same thing. You'll learn that saturated fats found in dairy products, meat, poultry, and egg yolks can aggravate inflammation from arthritis.

GLUCOSAMINE AND CHONDROITIN: A QUICK REVIEW
Treating OA from a physically active and nutritional standpoint makes good, solid sense, and using glucosamine and chondroitin on

a regular, long-term basis makes perhaps the best sense yet. Healthy cartilage relies on three basic elements:

1. *Water:* provides both nourishment and lubrication.
2. *Proteoglycans:* a component of the cartilage matrix, these large molecules surround and are present in cartilage fibers, lending resilience to cartilage, thus making it stretchable and bendable for ease and range of movement.
3. *Collagen:* which holds the proteoglycans in place.

Proteoglycans are crucial to healthy cartilage. That's where glucosamine comes in. Chondroitin acts as an adjunct to glucosamine by working to literally attract water molecules into the proteoglycan molecules present in the cartilage.

GLUCOSAMINE

Glucosamine is a building block of the proteoglycans. It is comprised of glucose and the amino acid glutamine. Without the presence of glucosamine, or if it is present in diminished quantities, production of proteoglycans is decreased and as a result there is less water drawn to the area. Glucosamine is so important to people with OA because it can do what some people call miraculous: help the body repair cartilage that has already been damaged or eroded.

In addition to jump-starting collagen production and even repairing damaged collagen, the supplement has been shown to reduce the pain associated with OA, and even give those with the disease increased mobility via improved functioning of the joints.

Glucosamine is available in the United States without a prescription and in the following four forms: hydrochloride, hydroiodide, n-acetyl, and sulfate. *Take note that people who have thyroid conditions should not take the hydroiodide form of glucosamine.* The dosage most frequently administered in trial studies of the supplement is usually 1.5 grams a day. However, you should consult a healthcare practitioner to calculate the dose that's perfect for you.

CHONDROITIN

Chondroitin makes up the other half of the powerful pair of nutritional supplements. While glucosamine is associated with production of the ever-important proteoglycans, chondroitin performs its magic by acting like a "liquid magnet" to draw lubricating, nourishing fluids into the proteoglycan molecules. To put it simply, chondroitin puts the stopper on the naturally occurring enzymes that can promote deterioration of the joint cartilage.[2]

Why is the fluid that chondroitin attracts so important? There are two primary reasons: it "pads" and protects the joints, and it is filled with nutrients that contribute to the health and resilience of the cartilage.

Where is chondroitin found? Mostly in animal tissues and especially in the gristle surrounding the joints. But don't be alarmed. You don't have to chew on animal bones every day to get the recommended amount of chondroitin in your diet. Fortunately, chondroitin supplements work very similarly to naturally occurring chondroitin. And, better yet, the substance has been found to be nontoxic. Some other very important vitamins for OA sufferers are:

ANTIOXIDANTS

Antioxidants are important components of your diet because they fight cell-damaging free radicals. Free radicals have been implicated in a number of diseases, including heart disease, cancer, degenerative conditions, as well as aging. The damage wrought by free radicals is also thought to contribute to the progression of OA.

Vitamin A/Beta Carotene

Vitamin A and beta carotene encompass the carotenoids, and both are important in the treatment of OA. These nutrients are crucial for bone formation, among other things, and are found in alfalfa, orange and yellow fruits and vegetables (think color!), fish liver oil, parsley, red peppers, spinach, turnip greens, asparagus, and peaches. The recommended daily dose of vitamin A for the person with OA is 5,000 IU.

Vitamin C
A diet high in vitamin C can help slow the progression of OA and alleviate pain. The vitamin is found in citrus fruits, berries, broccoli, beet greens, mangoes, onions, papayas, spinach, rose hips, tomatoes, turnip greens, and many green vegetables. The recommended daily dose is 500 mg to 4,000 mg.

Vitamin E
Often referred to as *tocopherol*, vitamin E is found in avocados, peaches, nuts, seeds, cold-pressed vegetable oils (such as safflower and sunflower), whole wheat grains and cereals, wheat germ, brown rice, eggs, sweet potatoes, dried prunes, legumes, leafy green vegetables (such as spinach), asparagus, peanut butter, and sprouted seeds. The recommended daily allowance is 100 to 400 IU.

Selenium
Selenium is a powerful immune-system booster. It is found in salmon, tuna, swordfish, oysters, shrimp, cracked wheat bread, and sunflower seeds. The recommended daily dose is 55 mcg to 200 mcg.

VITAMIN D
Research has revealed that OA can be affected—or even worsened— by inadequate amounts of vitamin D in the diet. While OA is mostly associated with deterioration of the cartilage, there is also evidence that the disease is related to bone density, and that people with "porous" bones (indicating a lack of sufficient bone density, which depends on vitamin D) are more susceptible to the progression of OA. Studies have shown that people who have OA and poor levels of vitamin D increase their risk of worsening (however, not causing) their condition. The recommended daily allowance of vitamin D is usually set at 200 IU, but those with OA may want to increase their vitamin D intake or their exposure to sunlight.

Vitamin D is found in fortified milk, dairy products, fish liver oils, fatty saltwater fish, liver, egg yolks, mushrooms, sunflower seeds, sweet potatoes, vegetable oils, sprouted seeds, and nutritional supplements. Sunlight also facilitates vitamin D production in the body. *However, vitamin D should not be taken in supplemental form without calcium, and it can be toxic in very high doses, so please consult your healthcare practitioner to find the best combination for your needs.*

BORON

This mineral works in conjunction with calcium to facilitate the development of strong bones. It also helps the joints stay healthy. OA has been shown to occur with greater frequency in regions where boron intakes are low. You should include boron in your diet every day, and you can find it in apples (with their skins) and cauliflower. The recommended dosage is 3 mg per day for adults.

BIOFLAVONOIDS

These substances are found in plant foods, and they are important because they assist the body in its metabolism of vitamin C and also help to build strong capillary walls. In addition, they help collagen form and maintain a strong matrix; prevent damage by free radicals; slow down inflammation; and promote the healing of athletic injuries. Bioflavonoids are found in berries, green tea, citrus fruits, onions, and fruits with a pit (cherries and plums, for example). You can also get them from eating fresh vegetables, whole grains, and seeds.

FATTY ACIDS

The following fatty acids are powerful inflammation fighters: alpha-linolenic acid (found in green vegetables and other plant foods); gamma-linolenic acid (found in evening primrose oil, borage oil, and black currant oil); linolenic acid (found in corn, sunflower, safflower, flaxseed, and soybean oils); and eicosapentaenoic acid (also called EPA, and found in marine fish and plants). Taking these fatty acids in supplement form, or getting them through the foods you eat, will help your body curb the inflammation of OA.

Remember that each of your food selections should support your goal of optimum health and well-being. Avoid foods that aggravate your OA and focus instead on those that are balanced, healthy, and may even alleviate some of your pain. Bon appetit!

CHAPTER EIGHT

The Mind/Body Connection

"Simply by changing your habitual vocabulary—the words you consistently use to describe the emotions of your life—you can instantaneously change how you think, how you feel, and how you live."

—BUSINESS GURU ANTHONY ROBBINS

USING THE POWER OF YOUR MIND TO
REDUCE PAIN AND DEPRESSION

The mind/body connection; mind/body medicine; mind/body healing. These phrases have enjoyed buzzword status in the alternative medicine field for several years, and lately they're working their way into mainstream, traditional medicine. We've touched upon the healing connection between our minds and our bodies through creative visualization and affirmations, but now we're going to show you in a bit more detail how the pure power of thoughts, feelings, and emotions can trigger internal physical processes that reduce or even eliminate the pain and stiffness of OA (and many other illnesses, too). We will explore numerous ways you may be able to use the mind/body connection for your own benefit.

Many people have an understandable negative reaction when they first hear about mind/body healing. Maybe they associate it with the few extreme sensationalists who, frankly, make it sound a lot like latter-day snake oil. Or perhaps they've just heard a few too many glib clichés about the power of positive thinking. As you read ahead, keep your mind open to new possibilities. Some things may sound a little bizarre to you, especially if you've relied on traditional MDs who rely so heavily on prescription drugs and surgery for most of your medical treatments.

The great news is that scientific evidence is quickly piling up that proves we have enormous mental power over our own healing processes. It's not just that we can help ourselves feel generally better by thinking positive, constructive thoughts. That's true and it's certainly important. But the mind/body connection takes "Accentuate the positive, eliminate the negative, and watch out for mister in-between" to a whole new and exciting level. And what's really terrific is that you don't need to rely on (or pay) anybody else to make it work. You can literally do your own mind/body work—and feel immediate benefits—all by yourself.

TREATING OA WITH ALTERNATIVE MEDICINE

In many instances, alternative, or holistic, medicine can complement the more traditional approaches to treating OA and might be able to help you along in your arthritis fitness and nutrition plan. Here's a quick summary of some forms of alternative therapies you might want to try.

WESTERN HERBALISM: This branch of alternative medicine uses the herb *devil's claw* to treat the inflammatory aspects of arthritis. But devil's claw should not be taken during pregnancy. Also, infusions of alfalfa and celery are often prescribed by herbalists as nutritional supplements for people with arthritis. Other substances that can ease inflammation include bogbean, feverfew, primula, willow, and aloe vera.

AROMATHERAPY: If you're feeling down or have low energy, try inhaling the vapors of geranium oil. Ginger and juniper oils can also be beneficial and may facilitate the release of toxins in the body. Rosemary oil enhances circulation, and its aroma can help you feel more energetic.

ACUPUNCTURE: Long known for its therapeutic benefits, acupuncture can be administered to treat inflammation and pain and to enhance mobility and circulation.

REFLEXOLOGY: In this mode of treatment, points on the foot are pressed to effect a physiological change elsewhere in the body. It has been successful in treating pain and inflammation.

MASSAGE: Extra care should be taken when massaging arthritic joints, but gentle pressure and movement can help alleviate arthritis pain and stiffness.

Other useful treatments and modalities include acupressure, shiatsu, and Ayurvedic medicine.

Mind/Body Basics

Even hardened skeptics regularly experience the most basic sort of mind/body connection. For example, you already know that simply remembering (that is, just *thinking* about) an embarrassing event often triggers the same physical symptoms—red face due to increased blood flow, increased heart rate, etc.—you felt when the embarrassment first occurred. The same thing happens when you think of a loved one (or someone you're angry with), hear a meaningful piece of music, or even get a whiff of certain odors or fragrances. Your mind triggers the emotional/physical reactions. And mind/body researchers find it very meaningful that the very same trigger (sound, thought, smell, sight, etc.) that causes an extreme reaction in one person leaves another person completely unaffected. You know the feeling: a sentimental song makes you misty-eyed while somebody else not only isn't moved but they'd like you to just turn it off. The point is that not only do mind/body connections exist, but we actually create many of the associations ourselves. Sometimes we do this consciously, but often we don't even know we're doing it.

Okay, you might well be thinking, getting teary over a tune is one thing, but what's that got to do with easing my pain? The power of your mind over your physical health is significant. Remember, the tune is just a basic example. Now consider the extreme:

Candace Pert, Ph.D., is the former Chief of the Section on Brain Biochemistry of the Clinical Neuroscience Branch at the National Institute of Mental Health. The following excerpt is from her interview with Bill Moyers for his landmark public television series, *Healing and the Mind.*

PERT: People with multiple personalities sometimes have extremely clear physical symptoms that vary with each personality. One personality can be allergic to cats and the other is not. One personality can be diabetic and another not.

MOYERS: But the multiple personality exists in the same body. The physical matter has not changed from personality to personality.

PERT: But it does. You can measure it. You can show that one personality is making as much insulin as it needs, and the next one, who shows up half an hour later, can't make insulin.[1]

The implications of Pert's research are literally mind-expanding. These people are actually switching physical diseases and allergies on and off instantly with their minds. One day—hopefully soon—scientists and doctors will discover how it's done so "normal" folks can do it, too. Meanwhile, the message is clear: Even though we're just barely understanding how to access and influence it, we do have much more mental control over our bodies and health than we ever thought possible. And in the middle ground of mind/body connections between reacting to a memory and switching off diabetes, we have gained insight into some effective ways in which *you* can make yourself feel better both mentally and physically.

DON'T FORGET TO BREATHE

By now you're an expert on what happens to you when you exercise. Specifically, increased oxygen in the blood. That increase results in reducing pain and promoting regeneration of cartilage in joints damaged by OA. Plus exercise raises your endorphins—you'll almost always feel increased energy and lifted spirits.

But let's face it: you're going to have some bad days. The ones where you simply don't want to force yourself to get up and start exercising, especially if you're in pain and feeling down or depressed. Other times you may be in a place or situation where exercise isn't practical. At such times, simply becoming aware of and controlling your breathing is a great and proven way to increase the oxygen content in your blood, and you'll get to reap some of the benefits of active exercise itself. We're not suggesting that if you breathe correctly, you can return to a sedentary life. But you certainly can breathe new life into your energy and spirits, reduce stress and anxiety, and it's a great way to ease into your more active exercises.

There are other reasons to learn simple breathing techniques including having control over the autonomic nervous system which, among other functions, regulates the heart, circulation, and digestion, which, in turn, could stem ailments or disorders of these functions.

There are many other specific breath-control exercises and advo-

IF YOU'RE REALLY DEPRESSED...

If your "down" feelings are persistent or worsening, by all means, don't hesitate or feel awkward about telling your doctor or other key support people if symptoms such as these persist:

1. loss of interest in things you normally enjoy
2. lack of interest in sex
3. irritability or blue moods
4. restlessness or slowed-down feelings
5. feelings of worthlessness or guilt
6. appetite changes leading to weight gain or loss
7. suicidal thoughts or thoughts of dying
8. problems with concentration, thinking, or memory
9. difficulty making decisions
10. lack of sleep, or sleeping too much
11. constant lack of energy
12. headaches or other aches and pains not caused by any other disease or condition
13. digestive problems unrelated to any other disease or condition
14. feelings of hopelessness
15. anxiety
16. low self-esteem
17. nightmares, especially with themes of loss, pain, or death
18. preoccupation or obsession with failure, illness, or other unpleasant themes
19. fear of being alone

Of course, it's normal to have some of these symptoms some of the time. And there may be other symptoms of depression. These guidelines aren't intended and should not be used for self-diagnosis—only licensed and trained medical professionals are qualified to render a diagnosis. They're just meant to alert you to possible problem areas if symptoms deepen or don't go away.

cates, and we encourage you to seek out those that work best for you. Yet, no matter which particular technique or techniques you use, the underlying idea is the same: Breath control is perhaps the easiest, most effective way for you to experience the mind/body connection and feel immediate and lasting benefits whenever you want them.

The following technique works well both for increasing energy when you're feeling sluggish or fatigued and, somewhat paradoxically, for calming down when you're angry or anxious. Once you get used to it, you can do the deep breathing standing or sitting, while walking, driving, or being still. But you may feel a bit lightheaded the first few times, so it's best not to first try it when you're negotiating traffic in a rainstorm or, say, walking a high wire.

1. Draw your breath in powerfully through your nose (mouth closed) for the count of four. Let your stomach expand (rather than your upper chest) as you fill your lungs as much as possible.

2. Hold your breath for a count of five to ten, whatever is more comfortable. This is the time when your lungs are absorbing oxygen, so gradually work up to fifteen if you can.

3. Exhale through your mouth to the count of eight, trying to completely empty your lungs.

4. Repeat steps 1 through 3 just a few times at first as you get used to the feeling. You'll find your own comfortable counting pace. Gradually increase the repetitions to suit you. And repeat the whole exercise whenever you feel the need.

Note: If dizziness is bothersome, you may want to add a step between steps 3 and 4 to slow down the whole cycle. After exhaling, count to four before inhaling again.

After only six or eight breathing cycles, the slight dizziness quickly gives way to renewed alertness and energy, and to the feelings of calm and inner well-being we mentioned earlier.

Andrew Weil, M.D., recommends a similar Relaxing Breath exercise that helps him fall asleep, and get back to sleep if he wakes up during the night. He recommends experimenting with it in situations when you are angry, anxious, upset, or when you're experiencing physical discomfort or pain.

THE RELAXING BREATH:

1. Sit or lie comfortably with your back straight, and place your tongue in what's called the yogic position: Touch the tip of your tongue to the back of your upper front teeth and slide it up until it rests on the ridge of tissue between your teeth and palate. Keep your tongue there for the duration of the exercise.
2. Exhale completely through the mouth, making an audible whoosh sound.
3. Close your mouth tightly. Inhale through your nose quietly to the count of four.
4. Hold your breath to the count of seven.
5. Exhale audibly through your mouth to the count of eight. If you have difficulty exhaling with your tongue in place, try pursing your lips.
6. Repeat steps 3 through 5 three more times, for a total of four cycles. Breathe normally and observe how your body feels.

This breathing exercise produces a pleasant altered state that gets better with practice. Dr Weil recommends doing this exercise to the ratio of four to seven to eight, ensuring that your exhalation is twice as long as your inhalation. Dr. Weil says, "It doesn't matter how fast or slow you count; your pace will be determined by how

THE BUDDY SYSTEM

If you tend to stick with things more when you do them with other people, you might consider finding someone to work out with. The purpose of finding a buddy is to keep you both on track—to support each other if one of you breaks your commitment to work out, or to be there as a friend and cheerleader when the going gets rough. Your buddy may or may not have OA, but should share with you a desire to become fit. Ask members of your family or friends or post a note at the gym that you're looking for an exercise partner and describe your schedule and the types of activities you want to do.

long you can comfortably hold your breath. Practice this exercise at least twice a day, preferably when you first wake and before you go to sleep, or just before meditating. After a month of practice, you can increase the number of breath cycles to eight."

LAUGHTER AND HUMOR

It's been a long time since Norman Cousins famously whipped a life-threatening illness by watching Marx Brothers movies and TV's Candid Camera. Since then, scientists and researchers have gotten very serious about the medical benefits of laughter. There is now evidence that laughter increases the heart rate, deepens breathing, improves blood circulation, and stimulates muscles. Laughter also helps manage or reduce pain. Just as in exercise, laughter releases endorphins and other natural pain-relieving hormones.

Laughter worked for David M. Jacobson's arthritis: "I used humor to literally get back on my feet after a diagnosis of severe arthritis. If you lose hope and are taken over by fear, you become helpless. If you use humor and focus on a positive outlook, you can

HERE'S A REMINDER OF WHAT THE ARTHRITIS CURE FITNESS PLAN WILL BRING:

• Less or complete relief from pain
• Improved posture and appearance
• Heightened libido and better sex life
• Weight loss that stays off
• Feelings of vitality, joy, and appreciation for life
• Better circulation and digestion
• Compliments
• A healthier heart, and so, reduced risk of heart disease and stroke
• Lower blood pressure
• Strength
• Nicer disposition
• A sense of control over both pain and life
• A boost to the immune system which means fewer colds, flu, and other common illnesses including cancer
• Improved relationship with yourself

get through anything. When the arthritis attacked, humor was my defense."[2]

And humor lightens up a lot of other ailments, too. It turns out that good doses of laughter lower blood pressure, reduce stress, aid digestion, and help you sleep. There's even clinical evidence that laughter increases your body's supply of virus-fighting T-cells.[3]

So how do you use laughter to heal? Dr. William Fry, a psychiatrist and leading expert on how humor effects health, recommends that you build your own "humor library" of funny books, videos, or whatever tickles your funny bone the most. "If you're having a bad day, feeling down and want to goose up your immune system," Fry said, "just go to your humor library and find the things that make you laugh."

DEALING WITH DEPRESSION

Let's say you're having a really bad day. You may say to yourself, "This OA is really getting me down. I'm depressed. I'm so depressed."

Well, maybe you're feeling pretty "down," but are you really depressed? That's an extremely serious medical condition and if you have the symptoms (see "If You're Really Depressed... on p. 121) that don't go away, then you need to get professional help immediately. However, you can radically change your emotional and physical states by the statements you make to yourself and others about your condition. Realize that, most of the time, you can choose to describe your state of health or feeling more accurately by using words that suggest healing options or solutions rather than leaving you stuck in a "downer" mode.

If you tell yourself you're depressed, what happens inside? Most likely, you'll feel even more down and discouraged. Because "depressed" to most of us seems like a dead-end, overwhelming, hopeless state that leaves you powerless. The next time you have a bad day, try to break down your physical feelings and describe them in specific terms. For example, are you feeling low energy? Maybe some pain, too? Maybe some stiffness? Are you feeling discouraged that the things you've been doing haven't worked as well as you'd hoped? Are you sad or grieving? If so, about what? Use this opportunity to write these feelings in your journal to explore them even more.

What you first called depression may well be a combination of several feelings. And focusing on the individual feelings rather than an all-encompassing label "depression" will help you find better solutions. You'll almost certainly get better suggestions from those who care about you and want to help you. For instance, if you simply tell someone you're depressed, they may feel unprepared or unable to help. But if you say that you're feeling discouraged because your pain and stiffness hasn't been relieved as much as you would like, you will have motivated yourself and enabled others to get to the root of the problem. Making these verbal distinctions (like between "depressed" and "discouraged") may seem a bit subtle at first, but try it. You'll not only be on the road to renewing your body but your mind as well.

VISUALIZATION, MEDITATION, AND SELF-HYPNOSIS

Creative visualization is rooted in the mind/body connection and can help you prepare for your workout. Just before you begin warming up, and prior to the swimming pool, gym, yoga, or aerobics class, find a nice quiet place and lie down for five minutes. (If you need to drive somewhere to work out, do this before you leave your house.) Get comfortable. Relax your body as deeply as you can. If playing certain kinds of music helps you to relax, put it on. Close your eyes, and envision each limb of your body as relaxed and pain free. Then, imagine yourself in the workout in which you are about to partake. Watch yourself warming up, only maybe in your mind's eye you'll be able to stretch just a little bit further than you can in real life. Then see yourself doing the main activity, for example swimming. Watch yourself immerse into the water. That may be through diving, jumping, or easing into it via the pool stairs. See yourself smile as you recognize the weightlessness you feel in the water. Then, picture yourself swimming with ease and grace. See your joints moving, and all that nutritious synovial fluid pumping in and out of your joints as you kick your legs. Feel the strength you are building in your muscles. Watch yourself reach the end of the first lap, and feel the increased beat of your heart. Listen to your breathing as it has deepened, but notice you are not gasping. Watch yourself through several laps, all the while recognizing how athletic you look and feel in the water. Then watch yourself get out of the pool, dry off, and take a deep breath that refreshes you and brings you back into your present reality. Take a few deep breaths.

If it's hard for you to imagine yourself and keep control of the thoughts in your minds eye, then simply focus on relaxing your body, and repeat your affirmations over and over. Squeeze in an image of yourself whenever you can: remember what you looked like and felt like at your healthiest, or picture what you would like to look and feel like in a year.

When you take five minutes out before your workout and visualize these things, you are sending messages to your body and unconscious mind that these states are what you want and that they can be achieved. It will prepare you for your workout, and represent the routine as a pleasant, rewarding experience. For those of you who find exercise especially difficult or unpleasant, creative visualization may help you the most.

Beyond the effects of creative visualization for your workout, it can be healing for your osteoarthritis. Health researcher Norman Ford recommends visualization to reduce arthritis pain "almost anywhere in the body."[4]

Meditation is another tool for tapping into the mind/body connection. But what is it exactly? According to Jon Kabat-Zinn, Ph.D., founder and director of the Stress Reduction Clinic at the University of Massachusetts Medical Center, "Meditation is a way of looking deeply into the chatter of the mind and body and becoming more aware of its patterns. By observing it, you free yourself from much of it. And then the chatter will calm down.... Meditation is a discipline for training the mind to develop greater calm and then to use that calm to bring penetrative insight into our own experience in the moment. From that insight comes greater understanding, and therefore, greater freedom to conduct our lives the way we feel would lead to the greatest wisdom and happiness."[5]

But what can meditation do for your health? Studies have shown that meditation can lower blood pressure, reduce cholesterol levels, reduce heart disease, reduce appearances of tumors, and control pain.

Meditation "frees the mind" and brings it to a state of "pure awareness," thereby allowing the body to heal itself. Several books and videos teach meditation techniques, but for the most effective technique consider contacting an experienced meditation instructor.

Self-hypnosis is an effective way to reduce pain. David Spiegel, M.D., of the Stanford University Medical School, researched the effects of self-hypnosis on women experiencing pain with breast cancer. He had the women rate their pain at intervals every four months. Over the first year, women in the control sample reported that their pain had doubled—from a two to a four on the ten-point scale. But the group that was trained in self-hypnosis reported a slight decrease in pain, so that by the end of the year their average pain ratings were less than two.[6]

But what is self-hypnosis exactly? Dr. Spiegel explains that, "Hypnosis is really just a state of focused concentration. It's like being so absorbed in a good novel that you forget you're reading a book, and you just get caught up in the story. We couple that with learning to control the way your body responds. So, for example, right now, you have the sensation that in the part of your back that is touching the chair, but until I mentioned it, you probably weren't aware of it. We call that 'dissociation.' You've put those sensations out of your conscious awareness. If you can do that with the chair, you can do it with pain. So people who are focused on one thing in hypnosis can often filter out many uncomfortable sensations. They can learn to transform the feeling into some other feeling, or just pay attention to a different part of their body."[7]

Visualization, meditation, and self-hypnosis can and do work for millions of people. But they do require more training, practice, and preparation than some of the simpler mind/body techniques we've discussed. If you think these might be for you, ask your doctor, health-care worker, or other member of your expert support group to help you find the right kind of instruction and assistance in your area.

SUPPORT GROUPS AND PRAYER/SPIRITUALITY

Does having OA sometimes give you a feeling of isolation? Of being all alone in your pain? Do you wonder how you're going to make it through the day, sometimes? If so, consider a trip to your synagogue or church.

The fact is, people who have strong religious faith or spiritual beliefs live longer, healthier lives than those who don't. Jeffrey Levin, M.D., of Eastern Virginia Medical School, reviewed hundreds of epidemiologic studies and concluded that belief in God lowers death rates and increases health. Across the board, in groups of different ages, ethnicities, and religions, among patients with very different diseases and conditions, religious commitment brings with it a lifetime of benefits.[8]

That doesn't mean you have to belong to an organized religious or spiritual group. But that's certainly a good argument for surrounding yourself with supportive, caring people who can assist you both physically and emotionally—and maybe saying a prayer or two along the way.

If organized religion isn't for you, at least consider joining a support group. Being around people with OA or similar health challenges can do much more than provide you with a source of help, comfort, fun, and distraction from your condition (although those are important. Dr. Candace Pert cites research on women with breast cancer. Those who participated in a support group with other women "...lived twice as long as women who had the same chemotherapy but didn't get together to talk."[9]

Regardless of your personal beliefs, and whether it's clergy or a colleague, it's important to get out there, talk to people, realize you're not alone, and tap into some of the greatest medication in the world: the love and compassion of other people.

EXERCISE FOR LIFE

Remember what we said about liking what you do or doing what you like? The Arthritis Cure Fitness Plan is a *lifestyle* change rather than something you do for a few weeks. Do the activities you enjoy and incorporate them into the The Arthritis Cure Fitness Plan. Maybe ten or twenty years ago you were an avid runner or hiker. You may still enjoy doing those things—you *can* do them, even with osteoarthritis. Make exercise, healthy eating, and positive thinking a part of your life through the Arthritis Cure Fitness Plan. Stay open-minded to new possibilities. Embrace new challenges. Don't let having OA deplete you of a rich, full, and fit life—take control. Remember, you have all the tools, and now the knowledge, you need to become the happy, healthy, active—and pain free—person you envision. Go for it!

Seven Guidelines to a Healthful Joint-Preserving Diet

THE TYPES OF DIETARY CHANGES that you make in following The Arthritis Cure need not be limiting or difficult to live with—although you may experience some challenges while modifying your usual routine. Remember: Anything new takes some adjustment, and eating better means living a better life.

Before making any type of health care commitment, you and your doctor should determine how much you need to change your diet. But even small changes will be a step in the right direction. Even if you're one of the many Americans who was raised on the standard meat-and-potatoes diet, you'll be pleasantly surprised at how easy and enjoyable our plan for healthy eating is.

A sense of balance is very important when evaluating your diet. Adherence to a too-strict regimen can prove to be stressful and counterproductive. If the majority of your meals are comprised of healthful foods, then an occasional hamburger or piece of candy won't hurt. But when too few "good" foods are consumed, the body doesn't have a foundation for health.

If you love to cook, you'll find great adventure in our suggestions. Perhaps you see cooking as a necessary evil. If so, there's something for you to learn as well. Whether you cook every meal from scratch, or put together an occasional meal when you're not going out or ordering in, the seven basic tenets of our plan will make you a more enlightened, better prepared chef and consumer.

Following are the basic guidelines to a healthful, joint-preserving diet. We've tried to state the basic concepts in seven, easy-to-understand components to help you better grasp the connection between healthy eating and relief from arthritis.

These seven components combine to help you create better health, just as the many systems of your body combine to function as a whole. More than just a diet, these guidelines (which have been established through research and clinical studies) will not only help alleviate the symptoms of osteoarthritis, but will also assist you in creating a personal foundation for good health.

1. EAT A WHOLE FOODS DIET:

No matter what your school of thought, health care professionals are increasingly recommending that Americans consume less fat, animal protein, and processed foods; and eat more complex carbohydrates, fruits, and vegetables.

A whole foods diet is a varied diet, filled with different colored vegetables, fruits, and grains; raw seeds and nuts; beans; and fermented milk products such as yogurt. It also incoporates fish, poultry, and soy products like tofu. Ideally, your diet should be lower in animal meats, fats, and cheeses, and higher in low-fat milk products.

Whole foods are foods in their natural state, unprocessed and unrefined. We're talking about complete, natural foods—those that contain all the beneficial nutrients that have been discovered and some that have not yet been discovered. It's the difference between eating a whole orange that still has its bioflavonoids in the pith and membranes, and drinking a glass of pasteurized orange juice which is high only in vitamin C. This is not to say that the glass of orange juice isn't beneficial; it is. However, by making simple adjustments to your diet, you can increase your natural nutrient intake many times over.

Whole grains are far superior to refined grains. When flour is refined, for example, more than twenty nutrients are all but removed. When it is then "enriched," only five or so are added back. Refined white wheat flour is low in nutrients such as vitamin E, copper, manganese, and zinc, to name a few. Some of these are needed for bone health, others to counteract the effects of arthritis medications. You will see frequent mentions of whole grains because these are the best possible sources of some nutrients. But we understand that changes may be hard to make all at once, so feel free to substitute a less "whole" counterpart on occasion. Our aim is to reduce your aches and pains, not to introduce new ones.

Refined white sugar is another example of a food that should ideally be eliminated in a whole foods diet. Its consumption depletes your body of essential vitamins and minerals. This type of sugar is considered a "stressor" food because it adds additional stresses to your body yet provides it with no benefit. Refined white sugar has no fiber and no nutritive value. This sweetener comes with plenty of empty calories, can lead to excess food intake, and contributes to weight gain. Eating refined white sugar is a poor food choice, and you will not find any in these pages. There are many sweet and delicious recipes you can make without using this harmful sweetener. Yet again, while white sugar does not contribute to good health, a healthy individual can eat it in moderation without compromising their diet as a whole.

These are some of the comparisons between a processed diet and a whole foods diet. The overriding purpose of a whole foods diet is to increase your intake of natural fibers and nutrients, and reduce your intake of fat and sugar. Additionally, studies have shown that people who eat a whole foods diet experience more enjoyment from

STOCKING THE SHELVES

One easy way to ensure that you have the right kinds of foods when you need them is to shop ahead of time. When you're hungry, you don't want to have to run to the grocery store or even worse, the nearest fast food stand. By filling your shelves with healthy, whole food products before you need them, you can increase the likelihood that you'll use them when it's time to prepare a meal.

their meals and are satisfied more quickly. This results in less overeating, making it easier to maintain your health and weight.

2. EAT A VARIETY OF FOODS:

When you eat a wide range of foods you give yourself the benefit of a myriad of nutrients. The standard American diet focuses on a narrow range of food choices: wheat as the grain, beef and chicken for protein, iceberg lettuce and tomatoes for vegetables. And while you may think you're getting a variety of foods in one day, if you're eating eggs, bacon, and hash browns for breakfast, it's the same nutritionally as a lunch of a hamburger and French fries or a dinner of a steak and baked potato. While these foods are fine—and even delicious—to eat in moderation, eaten routinely they limit our nutrient intake. Studies are also revealing that daily consumption of refined, processed foods can lead to a hypersensitivity toward these foods, making our bodies more susceptible to heartburn, gas, and indigestion, among other discomforts.

Our ancestors consumed a variety of foods by eating fruits and vegetables that seasonally came from the earth, and supplemented those with meat. As a result, different seasons yielded different foods and diets varied dramatically. You can vary your own diet

---

SEVEN GUIDELINES TO A HEALTHFUL, JOINT-PRESERVING DIET RECAP

1. Eat a whole foods diet. Basic, unprocessed, natural foods whenever possible.
2. Eat a variety of foods. Remember to eat a rainbow of colors.
3. Focus on inflammation-reducing foods. Avoid trans-fatty acids.
4. Choose foods high in antioxidants. Attack the free radicals, protect your joints.
5. Include foods high in bioflavonoids. Supplement your body with these natural immune boosters.
6. Maintain your ideal body weight. Do it for yourself and your health.
7. Replace nutrients depleted by prescription drugs. Up your intake of vitamins and minerals by juicing.

according to the season by shopping at local farmers' markets, where the produce comes directly from the growers. Also, look for lower-priced seasonal fruits and vegetables at your supermarket. You can eat well and save money too.

Experiment with spices, seasonings, and different foods. Many people like to experiment with exotic cuisines such as Indian, Chinese, Thai, Japanese, Mexican, African, or Middle Eastern, to name a few. Not only do these foods provide variety, but many of the seasonings traditionally used in ethnic cooking have healing properties.

Think of your plate as a painter's palette. Look for the brilliant reds, greens, yellows, and oranges of nature, not the browns and beiges of the major manufacturers. This is an easy way to get a broad sampling of nutrients without having to calculate the nutritional composition of every food. Remember, cooking and eating a healthy diet can be a joy—once you know the secrets.

3. FOCUS ON FOODS THAT REDUCE INFLAMMATION:

When there is tissue damage or over-use of a diseased joint in arthritis, the body's natural response is to send white blood cells to the affected area, causing inflammation. These cells produce prostaglandins and leukotrienes which in turn create a multitude of biochemical reactions. These are meant to heal the area, but also cause joints to feel stiff, warm, swollen, and achy.

Fortunately, nature always provides a remedy. Certain fatty acids in foods are known to counteract the inflammation response.

Alpha-linolenic acid (ALA) is found in green vegetables and other plant foods. This is an omega-3 fatty acid that blocks the specific kinds of prostaglandins and leukotrienes that cause inflammation.

Eicosapentaenoic acid (EPA) is found in marine plants and fish, especially fatty fish such as salmon and sardines. If you can, try to eat fish twice a week—more if possible. If possible, poach or broil fish because frying adds fat and destroys omega-3's.

Linoleic acid is found in corn, soybean, and other plant oils and is a precursor to EPA. It cannot be synthesized from other nutrients, but allows your body to make other fatty acids.

Gamma-linolenic acid (GLA) can be taken as a supplement, in black currant oil, evening primrose oil, and borage seed oil. These are also precursors to the kinds of prostaglandins that reduce inflammation.

Trans-fatty acids is a buzzword being circulated today that bears a lot of weight but has little meaning for most Americans. Simply put, a trans-fatty acid is a man-made molecule which may interfere with normal metabolic functions because their unusual molecular shape isn't readily recognized by our systems. Our cell membranes, our immune systems, and our overall abilities to heal are then compromised because an "outsider" has been introduced to the body, one that forces us to change to its rules, rather than one that adapts to our natural chemistry. Rather than contributing to the body's miraculous functions, trans-fatty acids are actually destroying them.

Trans-fatty acids can be identified on food labels which use "partially hydrogenated oil" as an ingredient. Many processed food products contain these hydrogenated oils, and the United States has recently insisted that all package labeling must measure and identify the types of fat in every product. To easily avoid these products, choose butter over margarine; olive and flaxseed oils over the many processed oils available; fresh vegetables over canned and processed ones; and make reading labels a part of your shopping routine.

4. CHOOSE FOODS THAT CONTAIN ANTIOXIDANTS:

One leading theory of what causes us to age is the free-radical theory. Free radicals are unstable molecules that roam about the body, attacking and destroying healthy tissue, including the tissue found in the joints. Osteoarthritis may be the result of free radical damage, and joint inflammation itself may trigger an even faster rate of new free radical formation.

Fortunately there is an antidote for free radicals: antioxidants that join with these unstable molecules and stabilize them, preventing them from doing more harm. Antioxidants are not at all new, just the old familiar vitamin A (and beta-carotene and the other carotenoids which are the plant form of the vitamin), vitamin C, and vitamin E, plus the mineral selenium.

Where are these antioxidants found? Most often in the fruits and vegetables that make up a whole foods diet.

Vitamin A and the carotenoids: Vitamin A is necessary for healthy cell growth, and is commonly considered the vitamin that gives you lustrous hair, clear skin, and good vision.

While vitamin A itself is found in animal foods such as liver and eggs, its precursor, beta-carotene, and the other carotenoids are found in plant foods. Beta-carotene also happens to be the pigment orange, so look for orange-colored fruits and vegetables when you shop for dinner and you can be sure you are including this antioxidant in your meals.

Vitamin C: This antioxidant is in many fruits and vegetables besides oranges. Bell peppers have higher amounts per calorie than citrus, although the many varieties of citrus make vitamin C a relatively easy nutrient to get. Cabbage (any color) is also an excellent form of this essential antioxidant, and its vitamins are shared whether the cabbage is raw or cooked.

Vitamin E: An essential antioxidant which protects red blood cells and is essential in keeping cell walls flexible and healthy, vitamin E is a nutrient lacking in most diets.

This fat-soluble vitamin is in short supply in the American diet because it's contained in

NEWS YOU CAN USE ON ARTHRITIS

The latest clinical research suggests that certain vitamins, minerals and nutrients are the most effective way of augmenting the effectiveness of glucosamine and chondroitin sulfates, as referenced in *The Arthritis Cure*. The following daily minimum amounts are recommended to keep the crippling symptoms of arthritis at bay*:

Vitamin A	**5000 IU**
Vitamin C	**500 mg**
Vitamin E	**150 IU**
Calcium	**300 mg**
Magnesium	**100 mg**
Copper	**1 mg**
Zinc	**5 mg**
Boron	**1.5 mg**
Chromium	**50 mcg**
Selenium	**50 mcg**
Manganese	**10 mg**
Silicon	**5 mg**

* They are discussed in detail in *Maximizing the Arthritis Cure* (St. Martin's Press).

the germ of the grain that is removed when refining whole grain flours into white flour. It's also missing in processed oils. For good health, eat whole grains and unprocessed oils. Asparagus and spinach are two excellent, delicious, natural forms of vitamin E.

Selenium: This mineral is considered the active partner of vitamin E, helping the body to utilize it. You can find it in sunflower seeds, swordfish, salmon, and shrimp.

A good way to increase your antioxidant intake is through juicing. See step 7 for more information on the nutritional benefits of juicing.

5. INCLUDE FOODS HIGH IN BIOFLAVONOIDS:

Found in virtually all plant foods, bioflavonoids are an essential tool in helping the body regenerate itself in a healthy way. They are essential for maintaining healthy capillary walls and metabolizing vitamin C, needed for building connective tissue. If you suffer from osteoarthritis, bioflavonoids can also be helpful by supporting your body's ability to manufacture collagen for the delicate connective tissue between your joints. Other important uses are:

GOOD OILS VERSUS BAD OILS

When oils are overheated and used for too long, such as in fast food restaurants, they become oxidized. Oxidized oils are loaded with oxygen-damaging free radicals (cell-destroying molecules). To counteract the dangers of free radicals, many doctors suggest supplementing your diet with vitamin and mineral supplements. You can protect your metabolic processes and cell membranes with antioxidants such as vitamins C, A (or beta-carotene), and E, plus the mineral antioxidant selenium. Optimally, you would get these vitamins and minerals through diet and higher doses (in the form of supplementation) are often required to fend off the dangerous by-products of chemically processed foods.

When choosing an oil to cook with, think natural. Olive and flaxseed oils are far superior to processed oils, and butter is better than margarine.

It's also better to cook with vegetable oils only at low temperatures. (And as you increase your "bad oil" intake, also remember to increase your antioxidants!)

- Preventing cellular damage from free radicals;
- Slowing the body's natural inflammation response;
- Preventing collagen destruction when the cartilage tissue is inflamed; and
- Speeding up the healing process of an injury.

Citrus is an excellent source of bioflavonoids, and is found in the pith and membranes of the fruit and in the central core. You enjoy the healthiest benefits of an orange when you eat it by the slice. Other excellent foods are green tea, berries, onions, and all fruits that contain a pit.

Bioflavonoids are also found in buckwheat (sometimes referred to as kasha). Instead of having a standard wheat dinner roll with your meal, cook some kasha, Russian style, with onions and mushrooms or try some Japanese soba noodles (also made from buckwheat) in a soup or a side dish.

6. MAINTAIN YOUR IDEAL BODY WEIGHT:

Let's be very clear that "ideal body weight" is not the same as the weight of movie stars and fashion models. Ideal body weight is the size and amount that is most comfortable and appropriate for your body. Keep in mind that there are many variables to weight depending on frame size and muscle tone.

If you believe that you need to reduce your weight to take pressure off your arthritic joints, you're probably right. So let that be your primary motivational factor. You can't manage your weight for someone else—do it for yourself and your good health.

The first step to remember when losing weight is to eat. This may sound silly, but skipping meals can lower your metabolic rate, thus slowing your body's systems down. This means that not only does your body not have enough fuel to operate properly, it also doesn't have enough energy to burn fat. Also, when you skip a meal or forget to eat, you're more likely to make poor food choices with your next meal.

If you are eating a diet full of nutrients (predominantly from whole, unprocessed, unrefined foods) your body won't have continual cravings for more food. Hunger is sated when your body is truly fed, not when you fill it with empty calories. Eat well, and your ideal body weight will start to reveal itself.

Of course it's important not to binge on fatty foods, but your body will ask for fat. When it does, give it healthy vegetable oils and oily fish products such as salmon. These fats can reduce the inflammation often associated with arthritis and will also satisfy your hunger.

It's also important to stay away from large amounts of sweets. Pouring these molecules of glucose into your system rapidly will trigger your body to store the sugar as fat. Sugar that cannot be stored as ready-energy turns to acid in the system. Your body wants to neutralize that acid quickly, hence the conversion to fat and hard-to-lose pounds.

Don't forget to exercise, even if it's just walking up that flight of stairs to your apartment or office. Exercise increases your metabolic rate and has the added benefit of stimulating the body to build healthy cartilage.

Remember that a weight loss of 1 to 2 pounds a week is the optimally healthy rate of weight loss. Don't be discouraged if your progress isn't that rapid. "Thin Thighs in Ten Days," is a gimmick. A healthy body on the other hand, is an investment of time and energy.

7. REPLACE NUTRIENTS DEPLETED BY PRESCRIPTION DRUGS:

Drugs prescribed for arthritis—primarily nonsteroidal anti-inflammatory drugs (NSAIDs) and other medications—can leech nutrients from the body. If you are taking any of these drugs, you need to pay special attention to your diet and eat foods high in nutrients you may be missing.

For example, many common NSAIDs (including ones sold over-the-counter) decrease levels of vitamin C in the body. Good natural sources of vitamin C are peppers, citrus fruits, and cabbage; whereas carrots provide an excellent source of beta-carotene, an antioxidant.

Juicing is an easy and efficient way to absorb the high levels of nutrients stored in fruits and vegetables. For example, it takes approximately five pounds of carrots to produce one quart of carrot juice. It would be almost impossible to eat five pounds of carrots in one day, but relatively easy to drink a quart of juice.

It's a good idea to have your physician or a qualified nutritionist measure your nutrient levels in the blood and tissue. Have a reading done on your levels of vitamin C, folic acid, phosphorous, zinc, and potassium. And, if recommended, eat foods high in these nutrients.

Another concern that goes in tandem with prescription drugs is the use of antacids containing aluminum or magnesium hydroxide. Often, these are taken to combat the stomach upset of prescription and over-the-counter medications. Yet, they can leech vital phosphorus from your body—one of the minerals necessary to keep your bones strong. You can counter this loss by eating foods high in phosphorus such as lean meats, lowfat milk and yogurt, soybeans, peanut butter, green leafy vegetables, oranges, nuts, and seeds.

Arthritis Cure Sample Recipe

Louisiana Gumbo with Okra

This soup is more like a stew. It is a perfect dish to prepare when the family converges and is in need of some great homemade food. Serve with brown rice in the bottom of the bowl or on the side.

$1/2$ pound fresh okra, washed and trimmed

3 tablespoons unsalted butter or extra virgin olive oil

$1/2$ teaspoon ground black pepper

$1/4$ teaspoon ground white pepper

$1/4$ teaspoon cayenne powder

2 stalks celery, quartered

1 onion, peeled and quartered

$1/2$ green pepper, seeded and quartered

5 cups fish or chicken stock, homemade preferred, or purified water

1 ripe tomato, quartered

2 cloves garlic, peeled

$1/2$ teaspoon oregano or thyme

$1/8$ pound andouile or keilbasa sausage, cut into pieces, chemical-free preferred (optional)

$1/2$ pound raw medium shrimp, peeled and deveined

$1/2$ to 1 cup shucked oysters and juice

2 scallions, pulse chopped or sliced

$1/2$ to 1 teaspoon sea salt

2 teaspoons lemon juice

$1/2$ teaspoon filé or sassafras powder (optional)

Lemon wedges

Hot sauce

Remove and discard the okra stems. Using a blender or food processor, pulse chop the okra coarsely. Set $1/2$ cup aside.

In a large stock pot, heat 2 tablespoons butter or oil and add all the okra except the ¹/₂ cup. Sauté on medium heat and add black and white peppers, and cayenne. Stir frequently, cooking until okra begins to brown, about 10 to 12 minutes.

Pulse chop the celery, onion, and green pepper. Add to the pot and continue sautéing for 5 more minutes. Stir occasionally, scraping the bottom of the pan.

Increase the heat, and add 1 cup stock. Cook uncovered, 5 minutes, stirring and scraping often.

Pulse chop the tomato and garlic, and add to the pot. Continue cooking, stirring frequently, another 5 minutes.

Add 2 more cups stock and continue cooking on a high flame, uncovered for 5 more minutes.

Add the remaining 1 tablespoon butter and 2 cups stock, and return to a boil. Add the oregano and sausage, and reduce heat. Simmer covered, for 45 minutes, stirring occasionally.

Add the remaining okra and cook 10 minutes.

Add the shrimp, oysters and juice, scallions, and salt. Stir and return to a boil, cooking for 1 or 2 more minutes, uncovered.

Add the lemon juice and give the gumbo one last stir.

Ladle gumbo into large bowls and sprinkle each with filé powder and serve with a lemon wedge. Offer a bottle of hot sauce, for those who like some additional heat!

YIELD: 4 TO 6 SERVINGS

HEALTHFUL HINT: Okra is high in manganese, an important antioxidant that protects bone and cartilage formation. Others sources of this needed nutrient are nuts, seeds, whole grains, and leafy green vegetables.

Updated Scallop and Shrimp Seviche

Traditionally, seviche is made with raw fish that has marinated for many hours in lime or lemon juice. The acid of the juices "cook" the fish without heat. These days it's not safe. Use our method of light steaming, and this recipe becomes a welcome light meal or appetizer—and the marinating time gets cut by 4 hours!

1/2 pound bay scallops

1/2 pound medium raw shrimp, peeled and deveined

1 cup purified water

Juice of 3 limes, 1/3 to 1/2 cup

Juice of 3 lemons, 1/3 to 1/2 cup

2 cloves garlic, peeled

1/2 red onion, peeled and cut in half

1/2 bunch parsley, thick stems removed and washed

1/4 cup extra-virgin olive oil

1/2 teaspoon herbal sea salt

1/4 teaspoon ground white pepper

1 head Boston lettuce

1/2 ripe avocado

2 scallions, trimmed and pulse chopped

Rinse scallops and shrimp in cold water and drain. In a medium saucepan, bring the water to a boil. Add the scallops and cover. Cook very briefly, just until the scallops begin to turn opaque, about 2 minutes. Using a slotted spoon, remove them to a bowl and cover with cold water to stop cooking. Repeat the procedure with the shrimp, cooking just until they start to turn pink, about 2 minutes. Remove to the cold water. Pour shellfish into a colander and drain.

Place lime and lemon juices in a medium nonmetallic bowl or container with a lid. Add cooled and drained shellfish, and toss. Make sure that the fish is covered with juice.

HEALTHFUL HINT: Avocados contain beneficial fat that lowers the LDL cholesterol (the lousy one) and increases the HDL (the healthy one). The fat in avocados is the monounsaturated kind, which is high in beneficial anti-inflammatory fatty acids. Here's a food that has fat that is so beneficial, it can be eaten often.

In a blender or food processor, pulse mince the garlic, red onion, and parsley. Add to the shellfish along with the oil, herbal salt, and pepper. Cover bowl and refrigerate for at least 1 hour. Stir after 30 minutes.

Carefully separate lettuce leaves. Wash and pat dry with a clean cotton towel; and refrigerate in a plastic bag to keep cool and crisp until ready to use.

Cut the avocado in half. Using a paring knife, score the side without the seed, in a crosshatched pattern, 1/2-inch wide. Slide a spoon between the shell and the avocado flesh, and scoop the pieces out. Add them to the shellfish mixture. Stir well. Taste and add salt, if desired (see Note).

Place several lettuce leaves on each individual plate, and scoop seviche into the center. Serve with slices of hearty whole grain bread on the side.

YIELD: 4 SERVINGS

NOTE: The avocado pit helps to keep the unused portion of the flesh from turning brown.

"I think that wherever your journey takes you, there are new gods waiting there, with divine patience—and laughter."
—Susan M. Watkins

Colorful Steak Fajitas

When you're trying to monitor your diet, the tastier the food the better. Look south of the border for meal inspiration.

Prepare the marinade, and marinate the steak for at least 2 hours.

4 cloves garlic, peeled

¾ cup lime or lemon juice, fresh preferred

6 tablespoons extra virgin olive oil

1 tablespoon imported soy sauce

½ teaspoon ground black pepper

One 1- to 1½ -pound flank steak, trimmed of fat

2 tablespoons unsalted butter

1 onion, peeled and sliced

1 red bell pepper, seeded and sliced

1 green bell pepper, seeded and sliced

2 plum tomatoes, cored and quartered

1 yellow summer squash, sliced

1 teaspoon herbal sea salt

½ bunch cilantro or parsley, pulse chopped

16 corn tortillas, warmed

TO PREPARE THE MARINADE:

In a blender or food processor, puree the garlic. Add the lime or lemon juice, 4 tablespoons oil, soy sauce, and pepper. Pour the marinade into a large, non metallic container with a lid. Add the steak, cover, and marinate for at least 2 hours in the refrigerator. Turn the steak over after 1 hour.

TO PREPARE THE FAJITAS:

When the steak has finished marinating, remove from the marinade, and pat it dry with paper toweling. Strain the remaining marinade and reserve.

Position the oven rack about 3 inches from the broiler heat source. Preheat the broiler.

Broil for about 2 minutes on each side; the outside should be

HEALTHFUL HINT: Red and green peppers, and tomatoes, are particularly high in vitamin C which is an antioxidant known to squash free radicals. Vitamin C is sensitive to heat and is easily destroyed by cooking or processing, so be careful when preparing this dish to keep the vegetables slightly crisp.

appetizingly charred but the interior should still be rare (so the steak can be later cooked with the marinade without toughening). Turn the broiler off, and proceed with the vegetables, leaving the steak in the oven.

Heat a cast-iron skillet or griddle and add the butter and remaining 2 tablespoons oil, making sure the fat coats the bottom of the skillet evenly.

Add the onion, and sauté over a high flame to brown the onion edges, about 3 minutes. Add the red and green peppers, and cook another 3 minutes. Keep the heat high enough to char the vegetables without cooking them all the way through. Add the tomatoes, yellow squash, and salt. Lower heat, and cook for 3 more minutes. The vegetables should still be crisp.

Meanwhile, remove the steak from the oven. Lay it on a cutting board and cut it against the grain into 1/4-inch slices. (Do not cut on the diagonal. This would negate the effect of tenderness to be gained by cutting directly against the grain.)

Raise the heat on the griddle to very hot, and add the steak. Drizzle 1/4 cup of the reserved marinade onto the steak and vegetables, at little at a time. If the pan is hot enough, the marinade should evaporate upon contact. Do not create a puddle of liquid in the skillet.

Place a trivet on the table, and put the pan on it. Sprinkle with the cilantro or parsley. Serve at once, right from the pan, with warm tortillas and other garnishes.

YIELD: 4 SERVINGS

"A complete lack of caution is perhaps one of the true signs of a real gourmet: he has no need for it, being filled as he is with a God-given and intelligently self-cultivated sense of gastronomical freedom."

—M.F.K. Fisher

Lemon Sesame Cookies

Unhulled sesame seeds are high in calcium and essential minerals. In this recipe they add a wonderful nutty taste and a crunchy texture.

½ cup unsalted butter, room temperature

1 cup real maple syrup or honey

Zest of 2 lemons, organic preferred

½ cup fresh lemon juice

1 egg, organic preferred

1 tablespoon real vanilla extract

½ teaspoon sea salt

½ cup unhulled sesame seeds

2 cups whole wheat pastry flour

½ cup oatmeal

2 teaspoons baking powder

HEALTHFUL HINT: Seeds and nuts are full of essential fats that are good for us, and these fats can also go rancid quickly. To avoid rancidity buy only whole, unroasted, raw seeds and nuts, and keep them refrigerated.

PREHEAT THE OVEN TO 350 DEGREES. PREPARE 2 OR 3 COOKIE SHEETS WITH PARCHMENT PAPER, OR GREASE WITH BUTTER.

In a medium bowl or food processor, beat the butter until smooth and soft. Add the maple syrup, lemon zest and juice, egg, vanilla, and salt. Beat well to combine.

In a heavy bottomed skillet, lightly toast the sesame seeds, stirring constantly, about 5 minutes. Some will pop out of the pan. Remove from the skillet as soon as they are toasted to prevent scorching.

In a large bowl, combine the flour, sesame seeds, oatmeal, and baking powder. Add the butter mixture to the flour and stir until moistened.

Drop teaspoonsful of cookie dough onto the prepared sheets, allowing room for the cookies to spread. Bake until the edges turn golden brown, about 10 to 12 minutes.

Using a metal spatula, remove the cookies to a cooling rack. Store in a covered jar.

YIELD: 2 DOZEN COOKIES

Gremolata

This seasoning mixture is a great way to accent a dish, without using salt.

2 cloves garlic, peeled

4 sprigs fresh parsley, thick stems removed and washed

1 teaspoon grated lemon rind, organic preferred (see Note)

1 teaspoon grated orange rind, organic preferred

NOTE: The skins of organic lemons are free of anti-mold agents and other chemicals, and they taste better.

Place the garlic and parsley in a small processor, and finely mince. Add the lemon and orange rinds, mixing briefly.

Sprinkle this mixture on sauce or gravy during the last 5 minutes of cooking. Simmer, covered, over low heat to allow the flavors to absorb.

Store in a covered container in the refrigerator, until ready to use.

YIELD: ¼ CUP

"So many sauces, so little time."
—David Dortman

CHAPTER 1

[1] "Slow Down Osteoarthritis with Diet Therapy" *HealthFacts*, Oct. 1996, v21, n209, 1(2).

[2] Ettinger, Walter H., Jr. M.D., M.B.A., "Physical Activity, Arthritis and Disability in Older People," *Clinics in Geriatric Medicine*, Volume 14, Number 3, 638, August, 1998.

CHAPTER 2

[1] "Osteoarthritis: Practical Steps to Successful Therapy," Gowin, Kristin M., Ralph H., Schumacher, Jr., Sept. 1996, v36, n9, 2048(6), Cliggott Publishing Company.

[2] Can Osteoarthritis be Cured?" *Tufts University Health & Nutrition Letter*, April 1997, v15, n2, 1(3).

[3] "Osteoarthritis," *Well-Connected Newsletter*, Report #35, August 31, 1997, Nidus Information Services.

[4] Barrett, Stephen, M.D., et al, *Consumer Health: A Guide to Intelligent Decisions,* Brown & Benchmark Publishing, 1997.

[5] Arthritis Foundation, Pamphlet #835-5440/3-96, Atlanta, GA.

[6] "Osteoarthritis," *Well-Connected Newsletter*, Report #35.

[7] "Osteoarthritis: Practical Steps to Successful Therapy," Gowin, Kristin M., Schumacher, Ralph H., Jr., Sept. 1996, v36, n9, 2048(6), Cliggott Publishing Company.

[8] "Can Osteoarthritis be Cured?" *Tufts University Health & Nutrition Letter*, April 1997, v15, n2, p1(3)

[9] Arthritis Foundation, Pamphlet #835-5515/1-96, Atlanta, GA.

[10] Theodosakis, Jason, M.D., M.S., M.P.H., Brenda Adderly, M.H.A., and Barry Fox, Ph.D., *The Arthritis Cure,* St. Martin's Press, 1997.

[11] Arthritis Foundation, Pamphlet #835-5515/1-96, Atlanta, GA.

[12] Arthritis Foundation, Pamphlet #835-5265/11-95, Atlanta, GA.

[13] Arthritis Foundation, Pamphlet #835-5265/11-95, Atlanta, GA.

[14] Theodosakis, Jason, M.D., M.S., M.P.H., Brenda Adderly, M.H.A., and Barry Fox, Ph.D., *The Arthritis Cure,* St. Martin's Press, 1997.

[15] *Ibid*

[16] *Ibid*

[17] "Can Osteoarthritis be Cured?" *Tufts University Health & Nutrition Letter*, April 1997, v15, n2, 1(3).

[18] "Osteoarthritis: Practical Steps to Successful Therapy," Gowin, Kristin M., Ralph H., Schumacher, Jr., Sept. 1996, v36, n9, 2048(6), Cliggott Publishing Company.

[19] "Overcoming Barriers to Successful Aging: Self-Management of Osteoarthritis," Holman, Halsted R., Kate R., Lorig, *The Western Journal of Medicine,* Oct. 1997, v167, n4, 265(4).

[20] *Ibid*

[21] *Ibid*

[22] Theodosakis, Jason, M.D., M.S., M.P.H., Brenda Adderly, M.H.A., and Barry Fox, Ph.D., *The Arthritis Cure,* St. Martin's Press, 1997.

CHAPTER 3

[1] *Fresh Start: The Stanford Medical School Health & Fitness Program,* The Stanford Center for Research in Disease prevention in partnership with the Stanford Alumni Association, KQED Books, 1996.

[2] *Fresh Start: The Stanford Medical School Health & Fitness Program,* The Stanford Center for Research in Disease prevention in partnership with the Stanford Alumni Association, KQED Books, 1996.

[3] "The New Thinking on Osteoarthritis," Clough, John D., M.D. et al, *Patient Care,* Sept. 15, 1996, 110-137.

CHAPTER 5

[1] "Developing an Exercise Program for the Elderly with Osteoarthritis," Olivo, Jane L., M.S.N., R.N., *Orthopaedic Nursing,* May/June, 1987, vol. 6, #3, 23-26.

[2] Kandel, Joseph, M.D. and David B., Sudderth, M.D. *The Arthritis Solution,* Prima Publishing, 1997.

[3] "The New Thinking on Osteoarthritis," Clough, John D., M.D. et al, *Patient Care,* Sept. 15, 1996, 110137

CHAPTER 6

[1] Francina, Suza, *The New Yoga for People Over 50,* Health Communications, Inc., 1997.

[2] *Ibid*

[3] "Play Away Aches: More Ways to Chase Away Arthritis Pain," Munson, Marty, Walsh, Therese, *Prevention Magazine,* Oct. 1995, v47, n10, 29(2).

CHAPTER 7

[1] Bellerson, Karen J., *The Complete and Up-To-Date Fat Book,* Avery Publishing, 1997

[2] Theodosakis, Jason, M.D., M.S., M.P.H., *The Arthritis Cure,* St. Martin's Press, 1997.

[3] *Ibid*

CHAPTER 8

[1] Moyers, Bill, *Healing and the Mind,* Doubleday, 1993, 182.

[2] "Laugh it off: The Integral Relationship of Humor and Health," Jacobson, David M., MSW, Health Beat Quarterly Magazine, Fall 1997, Djacob@flash.net

[3] "Laughter, It's the Best Medicine," Beaubien, Greg, Los Angeles Times Syndicate, Sept. 15, 1996.

[4] Ford, Norman D., *18 Natural Ways to Stop Arthritis Now,* Keats Publishing, 1997.

[5] Moyers, Bill, *Healing and the Mind,* Doubleday, 1993, p 126-7.

[6] Moyers, Bill, *Healing and the Mind,* Doubleday, 1993, 159.

[7] Moyers, Bill, *Healing and the Mind,* Doubleday, 1993, 158.

[8] "Reason to Believe," Benson, Herbert and Stark, Marg, Natural Health Magazine, May/June 1996, 75.

[9] Moyers, Bill, *Healing and the Mind,* Doubleday, 1993, 192.

American Academy of
Orthopedic Surgeons
6300 N. River Road
Rosemont, IL   60018-4262
847-823-7186
www.aaos.org

American Academy
of Osteopathy
3500 Depauw Blvd.
Suite 1080
Indianapolis, IN 46268-1136
317-879-1881

American Academy of Physical
Medicine and Rehabilitation
330 N. Wabash Ave.
Chicago, IL   60611
312-464-9700

American Association of Acupuncture
and Oriental Medicine
433 Front Street
Catasauqua, PA   18032
610-433-2448
aaaom1@aol.com

American Chiropractic Association
1701 Clarendon Blvd.
Arlington, VA   22209
703-276-8800

Ankylosing Spondylitis Association
P.O. Box 5872
Sherman Oaks, CA   91403
818-981-1616
800-777-8189
info@spondylitis.org

Arthritis Foundation
1330 W. Peachtree Street
Atlanta, GA   30309
404-872-7100
www.arthritis.org

Brenda Adderly, M.H.A.
323-932-0222
www.Brenda Adderly.com

International Chiropractors Association
1110 N. Glebe Rd., Suite 1000
Arlington, VA   22209
703-528-5000

International Institute of Reflexology
5650 1st Avenue North
St. Petersburg, FL   33733
813-343-4811
ftreflex@concentric.net

International Yoga Institute
227 West 13 Street
New York, NY   10011-7794
212-929-0586

National Chronic Pain Outreach Association
P.O. Box 274
Millboro, VA   24460
540-862-9437

National Commission for the
Certification of Acupuncturists
11 Canal Center Plaza, Suite 300
Alexandria, VA   22314
703-548-9004

National Institute of Arthritis and
Musculoskeletal and Skin Diseases
NIH Information Clearinghouse
1 AMS Circle
Bethesda, MD   20892-3675
301-495-4484
www.nih.gov/niams

Arthritis Cure Fitness Plan Journal

_____

_____

_____

_____

_____

_____

_____

_____

_____

_____

_____

_____

_____

_____

_____

_____

_____

_____

_____

_____

_____

_____

_____

_____

_____

_____

_____

_____

_____

_____

_____

_____

_____

_____

_____

_____

_____

_____

_____

_____

_____

_____

_____

_____

_____

_____

_____

_____

_____

_____

_____

_____

_____

_____

_____

_____

_____

_____

_____

_____

_____

_____

_____

_____

_____

_____

_____

_____

_____

_____

_____

_____

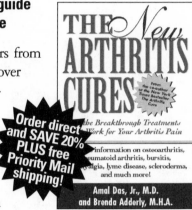

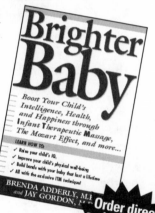

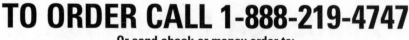